W9-CYW-713

The
Osteoporosis
Remedy

The Osteoporosis Remedy

Designing a Personal Prevention Program

Stephen Schettini

Avery
a member of
Penguin Putnam Inc.
New York

Every effort has been made to ensure that the information contained in this book is complete and accurate. However, neither the publisher nor the author is engaged in rendering professional advice or services to the individual reader. The ideas, procedures, and suggestions contained in this book are not intended as a substitute for consulting with your physician. All matters regarding health require medical supervision. Neither the author nor the publisher shall be liable or responsible for any loss, injury, or damage allegedly arising from any information or suggestion in this book.

Most Avery books are available at special quantity discounts for bulk purchase for sales promotions, premiums, fund-raising, and educational needs. Special books or book excerpts also can be created to fit specific needs. For details, write Putnam Special Markets, 375 Hudson Street, New York, NY 10014.

AVERY

a member of
Penguin Putnam Inc.
375 Hudson Street
New York, NY 10014
www.penguinputnam.com

Copyright © 2001 by Stephen Schettini
All rights reserved. This book, or parts thereof, may not be reproduced in any form without permission.
Published simultaneously in Canada

Library of Congress Cataloging-in-Publication Data

Schettini, Stephen, date.
The osteoporosis remedy : designing a personal prevention program / Stephen Schettini.
p.   cm.
Includes bibliographical references and index.
ISBN 1-58333-086-0
1. Osteoporosis—Popular works.   I. Title.

RC931.O73 L365   2001   00-048481
616.7'16—dc21

Printed in the United States of America

1   3   5   7   9   10   8   6   4   2

BOOK DESIGN BY MEIGHAN CAVANAUGH

I would like to acknowledge the invaluable contribution of Dr. Takuo Fujita, president of the Japan Osteoporosis Foundation and director of the Calcium Research Institute, who gave generously of his time and who impressed me as both a great scientist and a true humanitarian. Thanks also to Laura Shepherd, who edited the manuscript, and to all the staff at Penguin Putnam who made this book appealing and accessible to the widest possible audience.

The author dedicates this book to strong bones
and a healthy old age for all readers

Contents

The
Osteoporosis
Remedy

Introduction

I am a healthy forty-seven-year-old man. I work out frequently, eat carefully, and use nutritional supplements as wisely as I can. I'm tall, strong, and fit. I walk and hike a great deal and practice tai-chi regularly. The only thing that slows me down is a little arthritis and the occasional migraine. But when I was in New York with Dr. Fujita researching this book, I put my foot into a portable bone-mass scanner and got the shock of my life. My bone mass was way below average for my age. We looked at one another, then we did it again. Same result. Am I losing bone? How could that be?

Dr. Fujita wasn't that surprised. He shrugged. A little more, a little less—it doesn't make much difference. Like everyone else, the calcium in my bones is being spirited away, a few micrograms at a time. What about all the milk I drink each day? What about my lifelong passion for cheese? How could such a thing happen? I thought my worst problem was arthritis. Now the conversation takes an interesting turn. The arthritis is a symptom of the same phenomenon. When the body needs calcium for heart and brain functions, it releases so much of it from the bones that it swamps the body and starts to accumulate in places it's not wanted, like my creaky knees and aching hip. The key is to get enough calcium into the blood so that the body stops digging into its hoard. I want to live long, but not if my skeleton's disintegrating. Dr. Fujita promptly prescribed supplementation with active absorbable algal calcium (AAA Ca)—available in North America under the trade name AdvaCal.

Osteoporosis is a disease of aging. To put it another way, anyone who lives long enough will suffer from it. Although it is still considered by some to be a women's disease, it is clear now that men are just as susceptible. This fact is less apparent because fewer men live long enough to suffer the consequences. But our average life span is beginning to stretch into the danger zone. The emphasis on women developed for two additional reasons: First, women suffer dramatic bone loss at a relatively early age—the years following menopause; second, the most effective therapy devised so far—female hormone replacement—is only good for women.

Hormone replacement and other drug therapies take their toll on the body and carry certain risks. Many people like myself want to simply maintain bone mass and avoid the problem altogether, but this is not as easy as it sounds. Swallowing calcium is easy. Getting it into your blood and bones is another story altogether.

Bone loss is generally a very gradual affair. It begins at a surprisingly young age but doesn't cause problems for decades. However, once it becomes symptomatic the prognosis is not good. Bones weakened by osteoporosis break in a much more calamitous way than healthy bones. If you live long enough, your bones will eventually become brittle and break unless you take preventive steps.

Long-term consequences are very serious. Complete repair is impossible. Hip prostheses among the elderly are commonplace today, especially as more and more baby boomers reach retirement. They're keeping up their health pretty well on the whole, and may live to ripe old ages, requiring more serious attention to bone health. The only practical way to ensure skeletal health is to stop bones from becoming brittle in the first place.

There are several causes of calcium loss from bone. Age-related bone loss is caused not by an invading disease but by a hormonal imbalance in the body itself, which greedily and wastefully mines what seems to be a bottomless pit of calcium. The amount of the mineral it needs for metabolic uses is infinitesimal compared with the quantities stored in bones, so it takes what it wants with no regard for long-term consequences. But bit by bit, our sole store of calcium is used up. Our bodies are unprepared for the reality that we're living longer and longer and we need that calcium in our bones.

We all need calcium, and the safest and most convenient source is dietary. Calcium carbonate has been around for years, but it's only weakly soluble, so not much of it gets into the blood. Calcium citrate fares a little better, but it can only slow bone loss, not reverse it. A new form of calcium from Japan promises to be much more soluble—a combination of heated oyster shell and seaweed called active, absorbable algae calcium (AAA-calcium). Researchers claim it actually increases bone mass and has other metabolic advantages. Like all products described in this book, we look at the scientific evidence and tell you precisely what they can and cannot do. Because AAA calcium is an entirely natural product, it can be considered an alternative therapy. Because it has also been investigated in the most traditional of clinical settings, it has the credibility of a pharmaceutical product. This is complementary medicine at its best.

This book discusses the nature of osteoporosis and the latest thinking on how it evolves and what can be done about it. It accounts for the differences between men and women with osteoporosis. We go on to tell you when it will begin and how much time passes before it becomes symptomatic. We describe the scientific tests devised to confirm the approach of this crippling disease and then describe and compare various therapies in some detail. Finally we discuss prevention.

In short, the purpose of this book is to clearly and succinctly describe calcium, osteoporosis, and everything connected with it. (You'll be surprised to learn other things about calcium—for example, that it is crucial for the function of heart and brain cells.) Whether you suffer from osteoporosis or are just afraid of it, these chapters will help you understand your condition and what can be done about it. They will help you talk to your doctor in an informed way, and discuss various treatment options. We present all current diagnostic techniques and therapies—both conventional and alternative. And although some people lose bone more quickly than others, we all lose it, so we cover prevention in detail. Indeed, prevention is everything, especially if you're hoping for a long and mobile life. Finally, we describe ways you can keep bones strong and healthy with diet and, above all, with exercise.

The Osteoporosis Remedy shows how important it is to rebuild and maintain bone mass, and just how easy it is, too—as long as you plan ahead.

STEPHEN SCHETTINI

1

What Is Osteoporosis?

Osteoporosis, or porous bone, is a disease characterized by the loss of tissue from bone, causing it to become brittle and easily fractured. It most frequently affects the hip, spine, and wrist. Bone loss can start at a surprisingly young age and advance slowly, or it can accelerate rapidly following menopause, a deficiency of vitamin D, excessive use of corticosteroid medications, or a disorder of the parathyroid glands. In the absence of any such significant causes, bone loss proceeds more slowly, but it doesn't stop unless we take active measures to prevent it. The speed at which it progresses depends on the condition of your bone metabolism and the presence of a large variety of other risk factors. It is a silent disease, showing no symptoms until the first fractures appear, usually in later life.

Bone Formation and Renewal

Bone is alive. Far from being an inert mineral formation, this part of the body has its own structure and metabolism. Bone marrow at the center is embedded in a casing of porous, spongy bone and fed by nutrient arteries (many but not all bones have marrow). This light material is called trabecular bone. Although it is porous and not very dense, its structure provides great support. Trabecular bone in turn is encased by a thinner, harder, outer layer—cortical bone. Cortical bone is made of tiny columns of bone cells surrounding a central hollow with blood vessels, lymph vessels, and nerves. Covering the entire bone is a fine membrane of blood vessels and nerves. One might describe this whole structure as delicate. In fact it is one of the slowest changing parts of the body and is quite insensitive. But it's the strong, rigid bed to which our skeletal muscles are anchored, and the source of all locomotion.

Bone has four important functions. First, it makes up the skeleton and provides a rigid framework which, combined with our muscles, provides mobility. Second, some bone formations, such as the skull and rib cage, protect our internal organs. Third, the marrow found within certain bones is the body's chief manufacturer of blood. Finally, the skeleton is an invaluable storehouse of calcium.

The average-sized adult carries about one kilogram of calcium, mostly in bones but also in teeth and dissolved in small but crucial quantities in the blood. Like other body tissues, bone is in a constant state of renewal. Maintenance is carried out by specific cells—osteoclasts to remove old cells (resorb bone) and osteoblasts to grow new ones. When the process is in balance, bone maintenance is a very tidy affair. When bone cells reach a certain age they attract osteoclasts to the bone surface. The osteoclasts break down the mineral composition of the bone and release it into the blood, which carries it away. When the osteoclasts have finished, they leave a small hollow in the bone. This attracts osteoblasts that form new bone cells and gradually refill the hollow. This entire replacement cycle generally takes four to eight months. Bone is renewed in this way a few small areas at a time. It is an ongoing process, but not the only one that releases minerals from bone. Trabecular (spongy) bone is turned over at a faster rate than cortical (hard) bone. Children replace the mineral content of their skeletons every two years, adults every seven to ten years.

The action of osteoclasts and osteoblasts is controlled by the male and female sex hormones testosterone and estrogen, plus adrenal, thyroid, and parathyroid hormones. Don't forget this last one. As we age, parathyroid hormone increasingly mines calcium from the blood as if it's an inexhaustible pit, never considering that its natural resources may one day run out. You will learn much more about parathyroid hormone in later chapters.

Several disorders and disease processes may accelerate bone loss, such as vitamin D deficiency. But the process of renewal goes on relentlessly. In healthy children and adolescents, production of new bone greatly exceeds breakdown of the old, but after early adulthood—somewhere between our late teens and late twenties—the situation reverses. Osteoblasts continue to function and grow new bone, but bone loss overtakes bone formation. This shift increases with age. The long-term result is osteoporosis, which from this point of view should be considered a disease of aging, even though for a while it was seen as a woman's disease.

Osteoporosis is seen more often in women for two reasons. First, women live longer and therefore have more opportunity to experience the long-term effects of bone loss. Second, they go through a period of accelerated—sometimes precipitous—bone loss in the years following menopause, causing osteoporotic complications at an earlier age than men. Because estrogen replacement therapy has halved the rate of fractures in postmenopausal women, many doctors feel it is the best possible treatment for osteoporosis. But it doesn't stop all bone loss, and of course is not available to men. HRT simply stems the tide of bone loss for one particular high-risk group. Other contributing events continue to thin the bones of men and women alike.

How the Body Uses Calcium

Bone is made up of a protein framework upon which the mineral calcium phosphate is deposited. The protein is fibrous and provides resilience and strength. Calcium phosphate is a compound of calcium, phosphorous, and oxygen. It forms a crystalline latticework that makes bone hard and rigid. Calcium is available in many foods, particularly cereals, dairy products, eggs, and meat. Phosphorous is found in dairy foods and eggs, too, as well as in fish bones and green leafy vegetables. Deficiency of phosphorous is rare and is usually caused by kidney disease, a parathyroid dysfunction, a reaction to diuretic drugs, malabsorption, or prolonged starvation. Getting enough calcium, on the other hand, can be problematic. Children easily absorb enough dietary calcium to grow up, but adults find it increasingly difficult to get the mineral into the blood and hence to their bones. For various reasons this tendency worsens with age.

Calcium is the fifth largest component of the human body after carbon, hydrogen, nitrogen, and oxygen, the constituents of all organic compounds. It is the most abundant mineral in the body. Ninety-nine percent of calcium is found in bone, but the remaining 1 percent is distributed throughout the body. All cells—hormone-secreting cells, heart cells, liver cells, kidney cells, and brain cells—need calcium to perform their functions. The calcium used by cells is dissolved in blood, and is called blood calcium. Blood calcium accounts for only about one-thousandth of the body's total calcium content, but maintaining blood-calcium levels is a very high priority for the following reasons.

Calcium is essential for muscle contraction, the most important contraction being the regular beat of the heart. Low calcium levels lead to poor electrostimulation of the entire cardiovascular system and will quickly cause the heart to stop beating. Blood calcium is also crucial to proper functioning of the brain. Without it, nerve impulses cannot travel from one nerve ending to another. Our bodies respond immediately to the slightest decline in blood calcium by going on red alert, and promptly releasing bone calcium into the bloodstream. But most of the freed calcium is not used. It simply circulates in the blood. Much of it is eventually filtered out by the kidneys and passed into the urine but some is deposited in soft tissue and elsewhere, where it is really not needed and where it can even become harmful. The bone outgrowths characteristic of osteoarthritis—another slow but inexorable disease of aging—are one such product.

Types of Osteoporosis

Different types of osteoporosis are traditionally distinguished by the underlying cause, but usually more than one cause is operating. For example, women suffering from postmenopausal bone loss (caused by diminished estrogen levels) are also losing bone because of age-related shifts in the bone-renewal cycle. Various factors affect different people in different ways. Nevertheless, the following categories are widely used and they do help isolate and explain each different cause.

PRIMARY

Osteoporosis is said to be of the primary type when the principal disorder is within the bone itself or the bone-renewing cycle, as opposed to secondary osteoporosis, in which bone loss is symptomatic of another underlying disease. The following causes of bone loss fall into the first category:

Type I—Postmenopausal Osteoporosis

The hormone estrogen is an important stimulator of bone-renewing. Following menopause, estrogen levels may fall dramatically, and there is a corresponding decline in bone-building activity. Even after menopause, erosion continues relentlessly, particularly in inner, porous bone. The spine and the wrist are mostly composed of this soft bone and suffer most dramatically from hormone-related loss. In fact, postmenopausal bone loss in women is so fast it can lead to serious fractures within five or ten years. Because postmenopausal bone loss only affects women at a particular time of life, it is not the most common cause of bone loss, but it is certainly the most dramatic, and women at this time of life should be especially vigilant. For three to five years, some women may lose up to 5 percent of their bone mass per year. Despite this very troubling figure, many women exhibit no noticeable problem until the bone actually breaks or crumbles, usually in the spine or wrist.

Type II—Senile Osteoporosis

Aging-related bone loss is much slower than postmenopausal bone loss, but it affects hard outer bone as well as soft bone and often leads to hip fractures. This type of osteoporosis tends to cause problems approximately ten years later than postmenopausal osteoporosis and is the most common type of bone loss. Bone loss caused by calcium and/or vitamin D deficiencies also falls into this category.

Idiopathic

Idiopathic osteoporosis is a catch-all category for all forms of osteoporosis that we cannot clearly explain. Idiopathic osteoporosis is rare and can affect children and young adults. Sometimes bone loss occurs at the onset of puberty, a problem that could have dire consequences if not corrected. Fortunately, this often clears up of its own accord as puberty progresses. In adults, idiopathic osteoporosis is noticed only when bones break.

SECONDARY

Secondary osteoporosis is not primarily a bone disorder but usually the symptom of another disorder or the side effect of a pharmaceutical drug.

Polio

Poliomyelitis is caused by a virus that usually provokes only mild illness and is overcome easily by the immune system. Occasionally, especially in countries with high standards of sanitation and hygiene, the disease became epidemic. In its most virulent form it attacks the brain and spinal cord, leading to paralysis, loss of muscle bulk, and flooding of bone calcium into the blood. Such aggressive polio can paralyze the muscles used in breathing, leading to death. It can also remove massive quantities of calcium from bones. Some is excreted in the urine, but the calcium-saturated blood must dump the excess mineral wherever it can, usually in soft tissue. The kidneys attempt to remove excess calcium from the blood but can't keep up. This leads to huge kidney stones that may cause death by kidney failure. In countries with widespread vaccination, the incidence of polio is now very low.

Hyperparathyroidism

Overactivity of the parathyroid, a collection of pea-sized glands surrounding the thyroid gland in the neck, is known as hyperparathyroidism. Among other functions, the parathyroid hormone regulates calcium levels in the body. Excess levels of parathyroid hormone cause calcium to flood out of the bone and into the blood, leading to osteoporosis. It tends to deplete the hip bone most quickly.

Cushing's Disease

Cushing's disease results from another hormonal disorder—abnormally high levels of corticosteroid hormones in the blood. Corticosteroids are produced by the adrenal glands. The adrenals may suffer from their own malfunction or may be stimulated to release excessive corticosteroids by a pituitary malfunction. In either case, sufferers of Cushing's disease undergo a series of symptomatic changes including humped back, wasted limbs, skin disorders, osteoporosis, and mental problems such as depression, insomnia, and paranoia. Cushing's disease may also be initiated by excessive use of corticosteroid medications, widely used to treat rheumatoid arthritis, inflammatory bowel disease, and asthma.

Hyperthyroidism

Hyperthyroidism is a disorder of the thyroid gland that leads to general overactivity of the body's metabolism and, among other things, disturbs the body's calcium balance. Symptoms include weight loss, increased appetite, heat intolerance, and rapid, irregular heartbeat.

Paget's Disease

This is a bone disease common in middle-aged and elderly people. Paget's disease only affects certain parts of the skeleton, such as the pelvis, skull, collarbone, vertebrae, and the long bones of the leg. It directly affects the bone maintenance cycle by increasing levels of alkaline phosphatase, associated with the activity of osteoblasts, which form new bone cells. The result is deformed bone shape and inappropriate thinning or thickening of bone at various sites.

Multiple Myeloma

Multiple myeloma is a cancer of the bone marrow plasma cells. These are a type of white blood cell normally responsible for the production of immunoglobulins (antibodies), which fight off infectious threats. In this disease, the plasma cells proliferate and produce an excessive quantity of one type of immunoglobulin, while other types are underproduced, leaving patients prone to infection. This proliferation causes pain and destroys bone tissue, sometimes affecting the vertebrae and causing severe symptoms. Blood-calcium levels increase markedly and can lead to kidney damage.

Malabsorption

Many types of damage to and diseases of the intestines can result in impaired ability to absorb vitamins, minerals, and other nutrients. These may lead to a variety of ailments, including calcium deficiency and bone loss. The difficulties of Crohn's disease (a chronic inflammation in the digestive tract) and sprue (an intestinal disorder) are two such causes of malabsorption.

The Calcium Paradox

Dr. Takuo Fujita is a leading calcium researcher from the University of Tokyo who has published over four hundred and twenty studies on calcium, all in scientific journals. His years of accumulated knowledge have led him to formulate a new theory of bone loss and osteoporosis—the Calcium Paradox. The Calcium Paradox is a new approach to explaining bone loss and promoting bone growth. Several aspects of this theory are outlined below.

EVERYBODY LOSES BONE

Although osteoporosis may be triggered or accelerated by a wide variety of causes, everybody has one thing in common: Various processes of aging make calcium absorption and overall bone growth harder, and if we live long enough and do nothing about it we will all eventually experience net bone loss. Even those who have ample calcium in their diet may still lose more than they absorb, especially if they also eat large quantities of meat and salt.

Of course, some people are at much greater risk. Those who exercise little should be most concerned. They lose bone constantly, at a rate determined by their level of inactivity. Those with kidney disease, or women suffering the dramatic hormonal shifts of menopause may lose large amounts of bone very quickly. These groups must be monitored carefully, and must receive appropriate treatment. But even if the kidney disease is well managed or cured, and even if menopausal women follow a hormone replacement regimen, a less dramatic bone loss continues slowly and relentlessly, in them and in us. Where does it go? Why is it so hard to regrow?

BLOOD CALCIUM

Ninety-nine percent of all calcium found in the body is stored in bone. The remainder is distributed in the blood and soft tissues, some of it taking part in various metabolic functions. Despite this seemingly small amount—only 1 percent of the body's total calcium—the body uses it in many ways.

Quite apart from its presence in bone and teeth, calcium plays an essential role in metabolism. Although a humble mineral, it behaves in a hormonelike way, associating with proteins by means of calcium sensors that act just like cell receptors. Receptors are found on the surface of cells. They are like docking bays with a characteristic physical and chemical structure that attracts certain body chemicals to bind to them. Only specific chemicals can fit themselves into specific receptors, so this process is selective. Viruses also use this route to invade selected cells.

To regulate a metabolic function, the body releases hormones into the blood. These hormones bind naturally to the receptors of target cells and modulate (adjust) the functioning of the cells. The vast majority of body chemicals that act in this way are hormones.

Calcium is the only mineral that functions in this way. By binding with various body cells, it takes part in muscle contraction, the transmission of impulses from nerve endings to muscle fibers, and blood clotting. A decline in these functions quickly affects the heart and brain. Small fluctuations in blood-calcium levels can lead to poor electrostimulation of the cardiovascular system and can even stop the heart from beating. To prevent this and other problems, the body carefully maintains blood-calcium levels, mostly through the release of parathyroid hormone. Among other things, this stimulates the activity of osteoclasts (bone breakdown cells), causing calcium to be freed from bone and to enter the blood.

The key to avoiding age-related osteoporosis is to maintain sufficient blood-calcium levels to avoid excessive release of parathyroid hormone. Good diet helps—not just by eating calcium-rich foods but also by avoiding calcium-depleting foods (see chapter 2). Given the tendency of aging to increase bone breakdown activity and diminish bone renewal, this is easier said than done. Also, impact-loading and weight-bearing exercises (see chapter 6) are important stimulators of bone renewal.

THE PARADOX

Parathyroid hormone is the hormone responsible for calcium deficiency. A decrease in blood calcium stimulates the parathyroid gland to secrete this hormone, which removes calcium from the bone in order to maintain blood-calcium levels and facilitate such metabolic functions as heart and brain activity. Unfortunately, it floods calcium into the blood. The body then adjusts by excreting some of the excess calcium in urine and dumping the rest in soft tissue where it is both inaccessible to the skeletal system and an impediment to other bodily functions.

The paradox is that the buildup of calcium deposits in blood vessels is caused by the body's response to a calcium deficiency. Alzheimer's disease may be explained in part as another result of the Calcium Paradox. Calcium levels rise in the brain cells, and brain function starts to decline. Once again, this is initiated paradoxically by a calcium deficiency. The parathyroid hormone flushes calcium out of bone into the blood which adjusts levels by dumping the excess in soft tissue, including the brain.

Osteoarthritis is a joint disease characterized by cartilage degeneration and by the formation of bone outgrowths (osteophytes) that lead slowly to pain, stiffness, and occasional loss of joint function. Loss of calcium from bone leads to an increase of calcium in cartilage, causing it to degenerate, and exposing bone which then scrapes directly on bone with insufficient cushioning. The calcium also accumulates around the joint, forming physical outgrowths that restrict joint movement and increase friction.

A study conducted in Japan at the College of Nursing Art and Science confirmed that older women with the greatest loss of bone mineral density due to osteoporosis are also the group most likely to suffer calcium-containing plaque in their carotid arteries—the principal supplier of blood to the brain. Carotid atherosclerosis is a major cause of stroke, and this study is compelling evidence for considering it a calcium paradox disease.

Many researchers already agree that colon cancer is caused in part by calcium deficiency. Calcium enters the cell, then the cell starts to proliferate, divide, and subdivide until it becomes cancerous. There are many other Calcium Paradox diseases, like diabetes mellitus and some other cancers. As research continues, in time, the role of calcium in these diseases will be clearly identified.

Conclusion

Osteoporosis is a disease to which menopausal women are particularly susceptible but which affects us all. It is also an ailment of aging and will increase in incidence as the average human life span grows longer.

The body is engaged in a constant process of bone breakdown and renewal, but the balance between the two functions shifts in adulthood toward a net loss of bone mass. According to the Calcium Paradox theory, the parathyroid hormone is largely responsible for this bone removal but appropriate diet can maintain blood-calcium levels and prevent bone loss, and the right exercise can stimulate bone renewal.

2

When Will It
Happen to Me?

Are you at risk of developing osteoporosis? The answer is yes—if you live long enough. But there are many factors associated with bone loss, and different combinations of these factors place some people at much greater risk than others.

To avoid osteoporosis, you must evaluate your personal risk factors and understand which ones are contributing to your bone loss. Your doctor will help you with this and take into account scientific findings and other information that may not have been available as this book was written.

Those most susceptible of all are elderly, postmenopausal Caucasian women with poor diet and sedentary lifestyles, but if Caucasian men start to live ten years longer—which is exactly what's happening—they may well catch up. At the other end of the scale, African-American men who eat plenty of calcium and exercise regularly are less likely than anyone to suffer from osteoporosis, but as they live longer this statistical fact, too, could change. Low risk does not mean no risk.

In between these two extremes there are many factors contributing to bone loss. As long as the problem is addressed at an early stage, there is much we can do to prevent further loss and even to promote increased bone density.

Many scientific studies have tried to establish clear guidelines for risk of osteoporosis. On the whole they are extremely helpful, but in certain areas, the findings are inconclusive. The use of caffeine and alcohol has been associated in scientific studies with both bone gain and bone loss. While excessive use of coffee and alcoholic drinks is bad for many metabolic and physiological reasons, moderate consumption may actually be beneficial. Other risk factors, however, have been very clearly established.

Deficiency of vitamin D is an important cause of bone loss. Many types of cancers and especially multiple myeloma (a serious bone marrow disorder) can interrupt and destroy the bone renewal cycle. Other medical conditions contribute to accelerated bone loss that include prolonged immobilization, chronic inflammatory diseases such as rheumatoid arthritis, failure of the liver or kidneys, and any disease causing inflammation and enlargement of the lymph glands.

Bone depletion can also be caused by a class of rare connective tissue disorders in which the collagen type I molecule carries an inherited defect. Some of these are *osteogenesis imperfecta* (an inherited defect leading to brittle bones), *Marfan's syndrome* (an inherited disorder leading to abnormalities of the skeleton) and *Ehlers-Danlos syndrome* (an inherited collagen disorder). *Homocysteinuria* is an enzyme disorder that leads, among other things, to bone abnormalities.

Aging and menopause are the two most common risk factors for osteoporosis.

Age

The bone density we achieve around the ages of twenty to twenty-five is referred to as peak bone mass, because at this point the overall increase of skeletal mass tends to slow down and reverse. The greater your bone mass at this time, the better your chances of avoiding osteoporosis. The more you've got, the more you have to lose and the longer it will take for your bones to become brittle.

Most cases of osteoporosis are caused or aided by a gradual loss of bone mass that occurs for a variety of reasons. Over time the reduction of bone leads to the point of breakage, which is most often when osteoporosis is diagnosed—too late. Nearly everyone is susceptible to age-related bone loss brought on by the onset of secondary hyper-parathyroidism. Unlike primary hyperparathyroidism, this is not a disorder of the parathyroid gland. Rather, it is characterized by excessive secretion of the parathyroid hormone due to poor calcium absorption. Our increasing inability to absorb calcium results in the slow but constant leeching of calcium from bone. The bone removal itself is not unusual; osteoclasts are constantly wearing down old bone surfaces. The problem is, the bone-rebuilding processes of osteoblasts no longer keep up, leading to overall bone loss.

When osteoporosis is triggered by significant dysfunctions or disease elsewhere in the body—i.e., not in the bone itself—it is usually referred to as secondary osteoporosis. These forms of bone loss tend to progress more quickly than the primary forms of the disease, but still usually take years to reach a critical stage. If you are affected in this way, the disease-related factors of bone loss outweigh the age-related factors. But in general, the older we are the more bone we are likely to have lost. There are exceptions, most frequently among those who practice impact-loading or weight-bearing exercise regularly and/or those who have sufficient dietary calcium and are able to absorb it. Vitamin D helps the body absorb calcium, but with aging even its effectiveness diminishes. On the other hand, too much vitamin D has been known to intoxicate the body and cause bone loss.

The vast majority of people tend to reduce their physical activity as they get older, which is the worst thing they can do. Certain physical stresses directly stimulate bone growth. Also, as the skin and kidneys age, it is harder for the body to manufacture vitamin D, a key factor in absorption of dietary calcium. To top it all off, declining stomach acid levels after middle age make it even harder to absorb calcium. Indeed, the great challenge of calcium supplementation is getting it into the blood. It just isn't very digestible, and this problem increases with age.

As they age, advanced osteoporosis patients can be identified by an abnormal curvature of the back called *kyphosis*. People actually shrink, losing several inches due to the compression of vertebrae, which puts pressure on some of the larger nerves coming out of the spinal column and causes chronic pain. The saddest thing about this is that in most cases the osteoporosis was preventable, but is impossible to cure.

Gender

Women tend to be smaller than men and therefore have a smaller store of skeletal calcium. As adolescents, girls tend to exercise less than boys and begin to experience slight bone loss in their teens, whereas boys often continue to build overall bone mass into their twenties. Also, the larger frame and greater body mass of males place more stress on the skeleton and help stimulate the activity of osteoblasts (bone-growth cells).

But the greatest threat to women begins as they approach menopause. At this time, typically around age fifty, the ovaries begin to shut down and produce much less estrogen, the female sex hormone. As estrogen levels decline, bone loss can accelerate dramatically, especially from the spine. During menopause, a woman may lose up to six times more bone, relative to her size, than a man of the same age. After that time, her bone loss slows to match his, but by then her skeleton may be in danger of osteoporotic collapse, or close to it. And the bone loss doesn't stop—it only slows down. All other factors being equal, a man will reach the same degree of danger ten to fifteen years later, if he is still alive.

An even greater threat to women is premature menopause. Although this does not result in greater bone loss than midlife menopause, the early depletion of bone calcium leaves these women susceptible to fracture at an even younger age. They also have to deal with a weakened skeleton for a longer period of time and therefore usually experience more complications.

Obese women literally have an extra layer of protection. Even though the ovaries of all menopausal women stop producing estrogens and androgens (female and male sex hormones), androstenedione (a natural steroidal hormone) is produced in fatty tissue and converted to estrogen, reducing the bone-depleting effects of menopause. To a certain extent, more fat means more estrogen and less bone loss. Still, this is no reason to overlook the many health hazards associated with obesity.

Body Type

Body weight, body mass, and muscle strength are all directly related to bone mass. One of the main functions of the skeleton is to support the body, so it's not surprising that the bone-growth cycle responds to impact-loading or weight-bearing activity. The one bone-stressing activity we all have in common is carrying our bodies around, although this stresses some bones more than others, notably the hip and the bones of the upper leg (femur) and lower leg (tibia).

Greater body mass generally means stronger bones and more efficient bone growth. You may interpret this as another good reason to be fat, but too much fat raises the risk of much more immediate and dramatic dangers than osteoporosis—hypertension, stroke, and coronary artery disease for a start. It also adds greatly to the risk of diabetes and to the discomfort of osteoarthritis.

Nevertheless, slender or very thin people are at greater risk of bone loss, and if you grew up that way, you probably have less bone to lose. No matter what your age, increasing your weight will reduce your rate of calcium loss. A recent study confirmed that weight gain from the age of twenty-five upward is associated with a significantly lower risk of fracture. Weight loss is sometimes seen to accelerate bone loss in some patients, bringing them to the brink of osteoporotic fractures. For example, depression and/or poverty among the lonely elderly is often a cause of poor nutrition and weight loss, leading to increased risk of osteoporosis.

Ancestry

FAMILY

The age in life at which one's bone mass reaches its maximum seems to be determined at least in part by heredity. Some people will create less bone during youth and adolescence and, therefore, have less to lose. Unless they take steps to maintain or build bone mass, they risk early osteoporosis. The metabolic rate of bone loss over one's lifetime may also be inherited. So, if you have family members with osteoporosis, it would be wise to get your own bone mineral density checked.

In any case, studies show that daughters of osteoporotic women tend to have somewhat less bone mass than normal. Remember, such a predisposition to lose bone early and quickly is only one of many possible contributing factors. Whatever your overall rate of bone loss, other causes such as menopause (especially early or forced), certain drugs, poor diet, and a sedentary lifestyle will all play their part to inflate the figure.

A Los Angeles study of preteen girls reported in the *New England Journal of Medicine* showed that genes linked to vitamin D metabolism may help identify those at particular risk of osteoporosis. Dr. Vicente Gilsanz of the Children's Hospital of Los Angeles who conducted the study notes that bone mineral density is strongly controlled by genetic factors. Recent studies suggest that genetic differences in vitamin D receptors may account for inherited variability in bone mass. The researchers believe that by noting the type of vitamin D receptor genes a girl has, they can predict the density of bone in the lower spine and the thighbone. This study is still not definitive and must be continued using twins and families to produce unambiguous results. Even if this theory proves to be true, it is unlikely that this risk factor will outweigh all others, and most scientists still believe that bone density is determined by a wide variety of genetic and environmental factors, including but not necessarily limited to those currently recognized and described in this chapter.

Another study—this one from the Netherlands—studied the mutation of a gene that controls the production of the type of collagen involved in bone production. Dr. Stuart H. Ralston and his colleagues, reporting in the *New England Journal of Medicine,* found a consistent association between this mutation and bone density in the spine and hip. They concluded that DNA analysis should play a part in determining the risk of osteoporosis.

Scientists are far from discovering a single genetic cause of osteoporosis. And again, if it exists, it is unlikely to outweigh all other factors. If you are at increased risk due to genetic factors, you can balance the equation somewhat by minimizing other risk factors.

RACE

Statistics show that Caucasians, Asians, and Hispanics are at the greatest risk of osteoporosis. African-Americans tend to have more bone mass even in childhood, and usually have denser bones at peak maturity. African-American women generally lose bone at a slower rate than woman of other races. When their ovaries are removed prematurely—causing early menopause—their rate of bone loss is similar to that of the general population, so they are not immune. According to the National Osteoporosis Foundation, one in ten African-American women over age fifty has osteoporosis and another three are at risk. Nevertheless, osteoporotic complications tend to appear later in their lives than in the rest of the population, and they have more bone to lose before the situation becomes critical.

Statistical analysis of vertebral bone measurements show that African-Americans have shorter vertebra than Caucasians. But their inner, trabecular bone is significantly denser and it generally takes longer for bone mass to fall to critical levels. Because osteoporosis is a normal disease of aging, the lengthening life span of African-Americans will presumably lead to a greater incidence of this disease.

Another study reported that African Nantu women eat barely one-quarter of the recommended daily average of calcium. They bear nine children on average and breast-feed them for two years. They never suffer a calcium deficiency, seldom break a bone, and almost never lose a tooth. This report does not describe their longevity and long-term prognosis, but the case is interesting. While it is tempting to attribute their advantage to genetic factors, environmental factors may be the cause and more research is necessary.

Finally, we might see how diet affects osteoporosis by studying the native North American Inuit who inhabit the Arctic and near-Arctic regions. They eat more calcium than any other identified group—over two grams per day. They also eat massive amounts of animal protein and suffer more than almost any other group from osteoporosis. The high-protein diet itself may entirely explain the high rate of bone loss, since high protein intake has been associated with increased risk of bone loss. However, genetic factors could also play a role.

Menopause

Postmenopausal estrogen deficiency in women is often a cause of profound bone loss. Hundreds of thousands of women worldwide have received hormone replacement therapy (HRT) over the last three decades and have experienced relative bone mass stability, among other benefits. HRT has been so effective that for a while estrogen replacement was actually considered the primary course of treatment against osteoporosis. This approach was of little help to men, nor to the many women for whom such treatment posed too great a risk of endometrial cancer (cancer of the lining of the uterus). Women are now also supplemented with progesterone (the other female hormone) or a synthetic substitute to prevent uterine cancer. Although we now view the causes of osteoporosis in a much wider context, postmenopausal bone loss remains a serious, often dramatic, cause of calcium depletion.

A study by David Felson, a researcher at the Boston University School of Medicine, evaluated the threefold relationship of estrogen, bone mass, and breast cancer. His team found that women with dense bones are at greater risk for breast cancer. He explains their greater bone mass as resulting from greater-than-average levels of estrogen, an important factor in the development of breast cancer. This reflects another double-edged danger—that estrogen replacement therapy used during and after menopause reduces bone loss but may also increase the risk of breast cancer, although the connection between estrogen therapy and breast cancer remains highly controversial. A new medication, raloxifene, has been developed to treat osteoporosis while supposedly reducing the risk of breast cancer. It is described in chapter 4.

Menopause is the midlife period during which a woman's menstruation cycles come to an end. It is normally considered complete after the passage of one year without a menstrual period. Both estrogen and progesterone (female sex hormones) levels fall while gonadotropin (fertility hormone) and androgen (masculine sex hormone) blood levels rise. Diminished estrogen production in particular triggers many physical and psychological adjustments. There are also several metabolic changes, one of them being bone loss, particularly in the first two to five years of the menopause. During menopause, fat levels in the blood rise, increasing the risk of atherosclerosis (plaque buildup in the arteries), coronary artery disease, and stroke, so hormone replacement therapy against the ravages of menopause is attractive for several reasons. The trouble is, estrogen must be used with caution by women at high risk for endometrial cancer, and does not provide the same benefit to men. In fact, at the time of writing, none of the medications approved by the U.S. Food and Drug Administration (FDA) had been approved for use in older men. This reflects a temporary myopia, as sometimes happens in scientific circles, simply because of the statistical fact that many more women were affected than men.

Changes in estrogen levels are matched by changes in the bone-renewal cycle. The function of bone manufacturing cells (osteoblasts) is diminished while osteoclasts have a field day taking calcium out of bone. Trabecular bone, which is spongy and porous, breaks down more quickly than cortical (hard) bone. It becomes thin and gradually disconnected from its surrounding tissue, leaving the bone an increasingly hollow shell. The loss of trabecular support in bones leads directly to the weakening of the bone as a whole and its increasing dependence upon the outer cortical shell. Eventually it becomes so brittle that even a small physical stress can cause a fracture leading to irreparable structural damage.

The decrease in bone renewal is caused by decreased estrogen levels. The ovaries produce less and less of this hormone and progesterone during menopause. But that doesn't mean all woman lose bone mass. Androstenedione, a natural steroidal hormone, is produced in fatty tissue and converted to estrogen. Depending on how much fat a woman carries, she may have sufficient estrogen levels to ward off some or all menopause-related bone loss.

It isn't rare for the first signs of menopause to appear before the age of forty, though the mid to late forties is more common. Surgical removal of the ovaries before the normal age of menopause precipitates early menopause and early bone loss, causing the patient to reach critical bone-mass levels at an earlier age. Whether early or late, menopause causes many but not all women to experience hot flashes, sometimes for years. Under normal menopause, the time between menstrual periods becomes shorter at first, then longer. The hundreds of thousands of eggs with which a woman enters puberty have diminished in number due to aging. She has had approximately four hundred menstrual periods and the remaining unused eggs have deteriorated to the point that the follicle containing the eggs no longer produces estrogen and progesterone. Her hormonal cycles and menstrual periods are disrupted and she experiences all sorts of physiological and psychological disturbances. As she loses estrogen, she also loses bone, sometimes at an alarming rate. Unfortunately, the problem is quite silent until the damage has been done. Only years or decades later do unfortunate women discover the consequences of unbridled calcium depletion from their bones.

There are wide variations in the rate of bone loss among menopausal women. Some lose as much as 5 to 7 percent of bone mass per year for three to five years. Some lose much less. The estrogen released from fatty tissue does not fully explain the variations, and we do not yet understand all the reasons for this discrepancy. Calcium and parathyroid hormone play important roles, and there are probably other factors.

Estrogen replacement therapy holds bone loss at bay, but the rate of bone loss normally associated with menopause generally picks up as soon as therapy is stopped. Unfortunately, a large proportion of women who begin estrogen replacement stop it prematurely for various subjective reasons. In any case, although it dramatically prevents the symptoms of bone loss, it is not a cure.

The role of estrogen in bone renewal is only partially understood. Osteoblasts have been shown to carry estrogen receptors (a sort of docking bay to attract particular hormones), and so perhaps do osteoclasts. How the binding of estrogen to these receptors actually affects the bone-renewal cycle is still unclear, but it is undoubtedly a contributing factor.

In the most unfortunate women, osteoporosis sets in shortly after menopause. In other cases, postmenopausal bone loss is not too severe, but the gradual trickle of age-related bone loss continues. In a 1993 Australian study reported by A. H. MacLennan and his colleagues, a survey of 1,049 women revealed that only half of those with osteoporosis had undergone estrogen replacement therapy.

Increasingly, testosterone is being added to estrogen in hormone replacement therapies for women. As with men, this counters the effects of androgen deficiency—fatigue, lack of well-being, and diminished libido. In addition, it helps encourage bone growth (see chapter 4).

Men

STATISTICS

The number of men suffering from osteoporosis has always been smaller than the number of women—about one-fifth. The main reason seems to be the lack of opportunity for full progression of the disease. Osteoporosis starts later in men than in women, and men generally die before women. As the human life span grows longer due to improved hygiene and better diet, more and more men will encounter the complications of diminished bone mass.

For men who live long enough, osteoporosis tends to occur some ten to fifteen years later than in women. This is in part because men tend to grow larger bones than women. They also lose bone mass more slowly, and in a different pattern. First of all, there is no dramatic period of bone loss for men that compares with menopause. Second, they tend to lose trabecular bone in a less ruinous way. While in women the shrinkage is accompanied by a disintegration of the internal structure of the bone, leading to disconnected or perforated trabeculae, the internal structure of men's bones does not break down in the same way. The bone mass diminishes slowly, but the structure is not otherwise compromised until the total bone mass reaches critically low levels.

However, bone loss does gradually pick up speed. There is a definite link between age-related falling levels of testosterone, the male sex hormone, and rate of bone loss. Several other hormonal disorders can exacerbate male bone loss, including elevated levels of corticosteroids, growth hormones, circulating prolactin, or blood calcium. Hyperparathyroidism—elevated parathyroid hormone levels—also depletes bone. Secondary hyperparathyroidism, according to the Calcium Paradox, is a universal cause of age-related bone loss. This is not caused by a disorder of the parathyroid gland but is a response to inadequate levels of calcium in the blood.

Some unfortunate men begin to suffer from osteoporosis in their fifties or sixties. The first sign is usually back pain which can lead to vertebral compression fractures (structural collapse). The fact that these men in chronic pain are far fewer in number than women is of little consolation to them. However, many men suffer more than one such fracture before seeing a doctor. Do not be brave and silent about back pain. No matter the prognosis, waiting will certainly make it worse.

Men lose bone mass at about the same rate as women, but they have more to lose and it thins out in a different way. The hard shell (cortical bone) is depleted from the inner surface, but often regrows from the outside. Inside, trabecular bone thins evenly, widening but hardly disturbing the airy structure of this porous bone. Women tend to lose individual trabeculae (the building bricks of trabecular bone), meaning that its structural integrity is compromised without their having to lose as much bone as men. On average, men generally take a decade or so longer than women to reach the stage where low bone-mass density leads to a diagnosis of osteoporosis.

Dr. Sundeep Khosla, of the Bone and Mineral Metabolism Research Program and his team at the Mayo Clinic have found that bone mineral density corresponds more reliably to estrogen levels than testosterone, and theorize that estrogen deficiency may cause bone loss in men. So estrogen replacement may be an effective, though partial, treatment for male osteoporosis. In fact, the combined role of all sex hormones in both men and women is not completely understood and is still under investigation.

TESTOSTERONE AND BONE GROWTH

Although the role of testosterone in male osteoporosis is still unclear, there is no doubt that it plays a part in bone maintenance, a complicated role that involves estradiol (a potent estrogen). It is also known that testosterone replacement therapy improves bone density in men with hypogonadal osteoporosis (caused by low testosterone levels).

Low testosterone levels are an important cause of bone loss in men. Therapeutic replacement of the male hormones androgen and testosterone slows bone loss in many cases, and also improves libido and mood, among other things. The trouble is, testosterone replacement raises the risk of prostate cancer for men. In fact, the primary treatment for prostate cancer is a strategic reduction of these two hormones by chemical or surgical castration.

One of testosterone's functions is to stimulate bone and muscle growth, so when it is in short supply the bone renewal cycle becomes unbalanced. Testosterone deficiency is not an uncommon problem among men, though many are secretive about it. It usually becomes noticeable around age sixty and is marked by decreased libido, and sometimes impotence. This follows decades of slowly decreasing testosterone levels, during which bone discarded by osteoclasts is not adequately replaced by the bone-rebuilding activity of osteoblasts.

Testosterone levels can fall without necessarily affecting libido, and may in fact go unnoticed. So men who suspect or fear bone depletion—anyone in his seventies—should ask his physician to test for levels of this male hormone. Low levels are usually caused by a deficiency in the function of the testes, the pituitary gland, or both. Most therapies used against prostate cancer attempt to halt testosterone production, so patients undergoing such treatment should pay special attention to their bones. Supplementation with oral calcium and vitamin D can help.

Testosterone deficiency in men does not produce the same effects as estrogen deficiency in women. In women, the dissolution of old bone is accelerated by sudden estrogen loss. In men, the decline of testosterone levels proceeds gradually. But testosterone deficiency does slow down bone renewal. We have seen that while the effect is similar— net bone loss—the pattern and extent of the loss is quite different. Furthermore, diminishing testosterone levels do not affect the bone mass of men as dramatically as estrogen loss affects women.

Men also produce estrogen in small quantities. Some scientists suspect that testosterone may be converted to estrogen by bone cells, and thus help to maintain bone mineral density. Others feel that estrogen's role in the male is fundamentally unknown. Still, there is little doubt that both male and female sex hormones play a role in bone renewal in both men and women.

AGING

As we age, our bones become less sturdy. This is true for both men and women. In men, bone renewal slows. In women, bone depletion increases. The net result is similar.

Decreased levels of sex hormones as we age affect the bone mass of both men and women. Both male and female sex hormones are implicated in this process, for both men and women. As we now know, the most dramatic loss of calcium results from a sudden loss of estrogen in menopausal women. Many women who do not take hormone replacement experience a period of accelerated bone loss following menopause. It then returns to a slow, relentless trickle like that of men.

Women generally lose bone at a rate of 1 percent per year, and this increases to 3 percent or more during the years of menopause and after. For men, the figure is somewhat lower than 1 percent and there are no periods of sudden loss, unless provoked by illness or a metabolic disorder.

As healthy children and adolescents it is easy for us to absorb dietary calcium and grow bones. Unfortunately, as we age, the body no longer regulates and maintains bone-calcium levels with the same alacrity, and we are forced to intervene with the conscious decision to test our bone density and take concrete measures to prevent further calcium loss and rebuild lost bone.

The problem of bone loss can be addressed in part by calcium supplementation. The trouble is, calcium becomes increasingly difficult to digest as we age. It doesn't easily dissolve in the digestive tract it and has trouble getting into the blood, where it is needed to maintain blood calcium levels and preempt calcium retrieval from the skeleton. Some forms of calcium are more soluble than others. Calcium citrate is easier to digest than calcium carbonate, and active, absorbable algae calcium (AAA-calcium) is easier still. Nevertheless, it becomes increasingly difficult for both men and women to absorb dietary calcium.

The Sedentary Lifestyle

Lack of exercise, particularly weight-bearing stress, inevitably leads to weak bones. Especially, children who do not exercise adequately will reach a lower peak bone mass at an earlier age and begin to lose what little they have sooner than their peers. Sedentary children—and statistics point in particular to girls in North America—are setting the stage for long-term risk.

On the other hand, men who exercise appropriately at an age when they are normally subject to bone loss may maintain their current bone mass or even grow new bone. For women, the best time to exercise is before menopause, after which the benefits are more modest. A good strategy for both men and women is to reach peak bone mass at a later age, so that you have more bone to lose and the rate of loss is slower.

Impact-loading and weight-bearing exercise (see chapter 6) cause muscle contractions that stimulate bone formation. A whole-body workout is the best, but an important focus should be the upper and lower back and the abdominal muscles which together maintain posture, balance, and the integrity of spinal vertebrae.

Moderate exercise that provides a sufficient cardiovascular workout may not sufficiently stimulate the right muscles to initiate bone growth where it matters. Walking or running may partially protect the hip, since these place a healthy stress the lower body, but they are unlikely to significantly help the spine.

Some types of exercise, and certainly excessive exercise, can compromise many metabolic functions, including skeletal maintenance. For women, any type or extent of exercise that leads to menstrual irregularities should be avoided. The appropriate types of exercise are described in chapter 6.

Medical conditions that immobilize patients for long periods can accelerate bone depletion. Under these conditions, efforts should be made to minimize all other risk factors and to eat appropriately as much as possible.

The inactivity of daily life in a nursing home for the aged or infirm will certainly contribute to bone loss and worsen the condition of those with, or at risk of, osteoporosis.

Tobacco and Caffeine

It has been reported in some publications that smokers are up to two and a half times more likely to suffer vertebral fractures than non-smokers. However, recent scientific trials in Omaha and in Germany were unable to establish a definite link between nicotine use and negative changes in bone mass. Again, lifestyle factors may be responsible for the discrepancy. In any case, there are plenty of reasons to discourage smoking. Women smokers can have earlier menopause and begin rapid bone loss at an earlier age. Tobacco has dozens of harmful effects on the body, including an increase in the liver's breakdown of estrogen. This leaves all smokers with lower estrogen levels, which may affect bone loss in men too. Smokers also tend to weigh less, an additional risk factor for osteoporosis.

Statistics show that people with high caffeine intake have relatively low bone mass, but this may be due to lifestyle factors, including the substitution of coffee for milk and other calcium drinks. There is no direct evidence that moderate caffeine use adversely affects the bone renewal cycle, but if you drink a lot of coffee or tea, don't forget your dietary calcium.

Alcohol

Statistics show that people who abuse alcohol suffer reduced bone mass. Although this is not surprising, the reasons are still not understood in full. There are probably many. Alcohol may directly damage bone and does seem to interfere with the bone-renewal cycle. From a lifestyle point of view, alcoholics tend to eat poorly, which certainly contributes to poor bone condition. The negative effect of heavy alcohol use on the liver is well known. Poor liver function in turn affects the body's ability to metabolize vitamin D and leads to impaired calcium absorption. Also, chronic alcohol use affects the nervous system and makes long-term drinkers more susceptible to falls.

Heavy drinking affects the bone-renewal cycle by impairing the function of osteoblasts, responsible for bone growth. The bone-depleting action of osteoclasts does not seem to be affected. Heavy drinkers who quit using alcohol generally regain their osteoblast function, all other conditions being equal.

A study conducted in Barcelona, Spain, focused on a group of heavy drinkers with no significant liver disease. The lack of liver problems minimized the possibility that metabolic bone disorders were caused by poor vitamin D absorption. Researchers noted increased blood calcium levels and reduced levels of parathyroid hormone, suggesting that alcohol has the primary effect of removing calcium from bone and releasing it in the blood. However, they concluded that moderate use of alcohol does not seem to cause significant damage.

On the other hand, research by D. T. Felson and others in a Framingham, Massachusetts, study revealed that postmenopausal women drinking at least seven ounces per week (one drink per day) of alcohol had higher bone density at most sites than women drinking less than one ounce. They concluded that the alcohol increased their estrogen levels and this in turn reduced net bone loss. A slight but less significant advantage was also seen for male drinkers.

Another study by D. Hemenway and others showed that women over fifty who were both very thin and who consumed at least fifteen grams of alcohol per day were particularly susceptible to fractures. Thinness is already known to be a serious risk factor for osteoporosis, especially in women.

In spite of studies implying the apparent advantages of moderate alcohol consumption, the overall statistical picture shows that habitual alcohol intake is associated with decreased bone mass. Considering its general negative effect on metabolism, alcohol abuse (but not necessarily alcohol use) may combine with other risk factors to worsen imbalances in the bone-renewal cycle. Nevertheless, research results on this subject remain widely divergent and quite contradictory, some researchers reporting the positive effects of drinking on bone, others asserting the negative effects. It is important to clearly distinguish between alcohol use and abuse and to moderate its use. Although American cultural sensibilities often equate alcohol use with abuse, moderate drinking does not seem to be a significant risk factor for bone loss and osteoporosis.

Phosphates and Sodium

Phosphate is the second major component of bone, after calcium, and has an important place in our diet. However, the proportion of phosphates in our food affects the way both minerals are metabolized. It seems that excess dietary phosphorous decreases calcium absorption and lowers blood-calcium levels. Indeed, calcium and phosphorous interfere with each other's absorption and should be taken separately. Such a dietary imbalance is very common in North America, although its effect on adults may not be very significant. In children and adolescents, however, this imbalance can have a long-term effect. Many teenage girls, for example, stop drinking milk and take up soft drinks. A study from Boston shows that those who do have the weakest and thinnest bones of their generation. They are substituting phosphate drinks for a calcium drink. However, the greater risk may be the absence of calcium rather than the presence of phosphates.

Excessive sodium intake is suspected to play a role in poor skeletal health, but no studies so far have made a definitive link.

Diet and Food Supplements

Milk is the oldest and most common source of calcium for growing youngsters. It plays an invaluable role in bone development, and the amount we drink at that time of life directly affects our peak bone mass. A study in England measured the increases in bone density of eighty twelve-year-old girls who consumed an additional 300 ml of milk per day over an eighteen-month period. They had a measurable advantage over others and consistently produced more bone than those without the additional milk. Inadequate milk consumption in youth is an important risk factor.

Eating too much protein, particularly meat, causes the blood to become acidic. To neutralize the acidity, calcium and phosphorus in the blood binds to the acids, depleting blood-calcium levels and causing the body to release calcium from bone. The acid-bound minerals pass through the kidneys and into the urine. A report in the *New England Journal of Medicine* demonstrated that a very high protein diet produces high calcium content in the urine. How much of a real contribution this makes to the development of osteoporosis is not clear. To confuse the issue, a Framingham study of bone loss over four years in elderly men and women showed more bone loss in those with lower animal protein intake.

What about different kinds of protein? Vegetarians and vegans do not suffer particularly from osteoporosis. This may be in part because their diet tends to contain less protein than that of meat eaters. Certainly, the greatest difference between vegetarian and meaty diets is in the type and value of the protein they contain. Meat is one of the richest dietary sources of protein. You must eat a large amount of vegetarian protein to match the protein intake of a moderate meat eater. Excessive protein intake among vegetarians is less likely than among meat eaters, and probably lessens their overall risk of bone loss. Scientific studies are needed to assess the relative contribution to bone loss of animal as opposed to vegetable protein.

Perhaps those with very high protein intake tend to suffer because of the things they do not eat—i.e., that are bypassed in favor of protein. A diet rich in protein but low in carbohydrates is probably not a good idea. A Dutch study reported in 1999 by the American Society for Bone and Mineral Research concluded that pubescent boys and girls on a high-carbohydrate diet built greater bone mass, while those who ate a lot of fat did poorly. Certainly, the worst time in life for any sort of nutritional deficiency is during childhood and adolescence.

A report from the University of Pittsburgh shows that dieting may reduce bone density in the spine and hips. A study of 237 premenopausal women, about half of whom lost an average of seven pounds during an eighteen-month low-fat diet, revealed that "diet and exercise-induced weight loss was associated with a twofold greater rate of loss in hip BMD (bone-mineral density)."

Intake of vitamins A and K plus magnesium all affect bone density. Studies in Sweden show that vitamin A increases bone resorption (removal of bone cells by osteoclasts), suggesting that high levels of this nutrient may increase the risk of osteoporosis. Vitamin A is found in liver; fish-liver oils; egg yolks; milk and dairy products; margarine; fruits like oranges, plums, and peaches; and vegetables like carrots. Vitamin A supplementation is rarely necessary and may be unwise.

A Framingham study showed that deficiency of vitamin K

impedes the metabolism of bone and increases the risk of osteoporosis. Vitamin K is found in green, leafy vegetables, especially cabbage; broccoli, and turnip greens; vegetable oils; egg yolks; cheese; pork; and liver.

Vitamin D deficiency in children causes rickets, resulting in the softening and weakening of bones. Childhood is the worst time to retard or damage the development of the skeleton and, even after recovery, these children may suffer accelerated bone loss and early osteoporosis. In adults, rickets is sometimes found among people with malabsorption disorders (difficulty absorbing nutrients) and also among vegetarians who do not consume milk products. Very occasionally, lactose-intolerant individuals may be unable to absorb their dietary vitamin D.

A report published in the *Annals of Internal Medicine* in 1977 found that patients suffering from osteoporosis were worsening their condition by taking too much calcium and vitamin D from over-the-counter supplements. Their problem wasn't the calcium, since calcium has no known side effects, except constipation, when taken in very large doses. The problem was toxic levels of vitamin D. Excessive intake of this vitamin upsets the metabolic balance of calcium and phosphates, leading to hypercalcemia—too much blood calcium. This is the last problem you need if you already have osteoporosis. The body responds by passing the calcium in large quantities into the urine, after which blood calcium levels fall, only to be replenished again when calcium is taken from bones. Not all the calcium ends up in urine. Another effect of hypercalcemia is the deposit of calcium in the fatty plaque that accumulates in soft tissue, leading to a variety of Calcium Paradox diseases such as osteoarthritis. Simply counting the value of vitamin D supplements is not enough. You must include your dietary sources. Vitamin D is found in liver; egg yolk; margarine; cod-liver oil; and oily fish such as sardines, herring, salmon, and tuna. It is also frequently added to milk.

Magnesium is an important component of bone, and low levels of dietary magnesium are suspected to contribute to bone loss. However, apart from some statistical research implying the possible slight advantage of calcium-magnesium supplementation, there is little data to support this hypothesis.

Fluoride is added to the water supply in many countries to prevent tooth decay. It can also cause a painful bone disease called fluorosis, which increases the number of osteoblasts and causes bone to abnormally increase in density. While some doctors feel that fluoride may be a useful way to strengthen bones, others are wary. Fluoride's role in bone maintenance is unclear, and while a little may help grow bone, the effects are questionable. An excess of fluoride produces mottled teeth, abnormal bone, and neurological problems. In laboratory tests of fluoride-initiated bone growth, bones continued to fracture in spite of dramatic increases in density.

The same study in Japan that revealed the connection between osteoporosis and stroke also revealed an important discovery about vitamin D. The lower an individual's levels of vitamin D, the more likely that calcium will accumulate in fatty plaque in the coronary arteries. Commenting on these findings, the lead author of the medical journal *Circulation,* Dr. Karol Watson, was surprised. He expected that since low vitamin D levels result in lower levels of bone calcification, they would also lead to lower levels of calcium deposit in arterial plaques. These finding are consistent with the Calcium Paradox theory, mentioned in chapter 1 and described in chapter 5.

Pharmaceutical Drugs

Most pharmaceutical drugs have side effects. Some of them are unfavorable to the bone-renewal cycle. However, you should not stop taking a medication simply because it is listed in this section. Consult your physician first. Good general practitioners are skilled at balancing the risk of combining various lifestyle factors, diet, and medications, and should prevent you from compromising your overall health. Nobody likes side effects, but some of these drugs are lifesavers.

Steroids, thyroid hormone, GNRH analogs, LHRH-agonists, anticonvulsants, and anticoagulants can all affect the bone-renewal cycle in a negative way. These are explained below.

STEROIDS

Steroids are a group of drugs that resemble biological hormones. There are two classes. The first, anabolic steroids, produce a protein-building effect like testosterone and other male hormones. Their abuse by some athletes is well known. The second, corticosteroids, are hormones produced by the adrenal glands. They contribute the greatest risk to bones because they are used extensively in many medical treatments, especially for inflammatory and skin conditions. Corticosteroid medications include cortisone, prednisone, prednisolone, and dexamethasone, all sold under a variety of trade names by many manufacturers.

Corticosteroids are effective lifesavers for people suffering from rheumatoid arthritis (severe, chronic inflammation of joints), systemic lupus erythematosus (chronic inflammation of the connective tissue that holds body structures together), and severe asthma (breathlessness), most of whom take a low but constant dose of steroids to control their condition. They are also used against other inflammatory, noninfectious diseases such as inflammatory bowel disease (chronic intestinal inflammation) and multiple sclerosis (a progressive disease of the nervous system) and are the only effective way to control a wide variety of skin conditions.

A study by Dr. Stavros Manolagas of the University of Arkansas conducted laboratory tests on the long-term effects of steroid medications. The researchers showed that corticosteroid drugs cause premature death of osteoblasts—the body's bone-manufacturing cells. They described the effect of steroids on bone cells as "devastating," and reported a threefold increase in the death of osteoblasts.

Recent research has come up with a stopgap solution to this problem. By taking the medication alendronate (see chapter 4) together with steroid therapy, it seems that such accelerated bone loss can be halted. Dr. Kenneth Saag of the University of Iowa studied the use of alendronate in 477 steroid users who also took calcium and vitamin D supplements. It was found that those using alendronate increased their average bone density during the therapy.

Alendronate is a pharmaceutical drug and has its own side effects, namely problems in the upper gastrointestinal tract, although few serious cases have been reported. Many doctors would consider the additional side effects of alendronate to be justified by the elimination of a much more troubling side effect—the severe bone-thinning action of corticosteroids.

THYROID HORMONES

Thyroid hormones include the pharmaceutical drugs levothyroxine, liothyronine, and liotrix, sold under many trade names by a variety of manufacturers. These medications are used to treat underactivity, swelling, or cancer of the thyroid gland. Dosage is set individually, and determining precise requirements for each patient takes a little trial and error. During this period of adjustment, the patient may suffer symptoms of thyroid overactivity, worsened angina, or congestive heart failure. Under no circumstances should you stop taking thyroid hormones just because you are afraid of osteoporosis. However, careful attention to other risk factors is important. Your physician will help you evaluate your total risk and devise appropriate therapies.

GNRH ANALOGS

Gonadotropin-releasing hormone (GNRH) agonists are synthetic hormones that resemble those released by the hypothalamus gland in the brain. They are used in women to control endometriosis (displacement and growth of uterine lining tissue to the pelvic region and elsewhere), uterine fibroids (benign tumors in the uterus), and other diseases. They work by inducing the ovaries to temporarily fail, causing estrogen levels to plummet. These low levels last only as long as the treatment, but the treatment must be relatively long—six months is not uncommon. Bone is lost during treatment, though it is apparently somewhat restored after treatment ceases.

LHRH AGONISTS

Luteinizing hormone releasing hormone (LHRH) agonists are used in men to treat prostate cancer. By affecting the pituitary gland in the brain, they cause the testicles to slow or shut down production of testosterone. The treatment is known as chemical castration and is much preferable to actual castration, which is sometimes performed. Its negative effect on bone is consistent with what we know about the role of testosterone in the bone-renewal cycle. Because of the risk of low testosterone levels, as well as the treatment's negative effect upon the patient's libido and morale, a recent approach to prostate cancer has become widely used. Called "watchful waiting," it uses no medication or intervention at all, but patients are monitored frequently.

Prostate cancer is very common among elderly men but is also one of the slowest growing of all cancers, and is often contained within the prostate without spreading to other sites. Many men have prostate cancer without symptoms and manage well without medication. As long as the cancer does not flare up, treatment is withheld. This results in a better quality of life and, of course, lessened risk of bone loss. LHRH agonists do not cure prostate cancer—they stabilize or slow its growth, at best. Since it is confirmed that prostate cancer can remain relatively inactive for long periods, the disadvantages of chemical castration outweigh the dangers of allowing the body to manufacture testosterone.

OTHER MEDICATIONS

The most important medications with bone-thinning side effects have already been described above. This section lists others that generally pose a less significant risk. However, when combined with other risk factors these drugs may tip the balance.

Potassium-sparing diuretic pills are used to remove excess water from the body by increasing urination and can lead to potassium deficiency, a risk factor in itself for bone loss.

Heparin, an anticoagulant, is used to prevent and treat abnormal blood clotting. One of its possible side effects is aching bone and bone loss. This drug is rarely prescribed in large doses or for long periods, but when it is, it should be considered a significant risk. Under normal conditions, the risk is minimal.

Methotrexate is used to treat lymphoma (cancer of the lymph nodes), leukemia (cancer of white blood cells), and other cancers. It has also been used against psoriasis, a skin condition, and rheumatoid arthritis, both chronic inflammatory conditions requiring long-term medication. Since it is commonly used in large doses and for long periods, it can potentially be a significant risk factor. However, its intervention is usually urgent and the disadvantages of temporary bone loss are far outweighed by the need to fight cancer.

Lithium is used to treat mania and manic depression. One of its side effects is increased production of parathyroid hormone, which removes calcium from bone.

A variety of anticonvulsants and other drugs used to prevent seizures may interfere with calcium absorption and vitamin D production by stimulating parathyroid activity.

Antacids contain aluminum, an element of no known value to the body and one that removes calcium from the blood and passes it into the urine. Low blood-calcium levels then stimulate the release of parathyroid hormone, which replenishes blood calcium from skeletal stores.

Removal of the thyroid gland can also cause bone loss. The thyroid makes calcitonin (see chapter 4), a hormone that helps control blood calcium levels by slowing bone loss, and its removal may adversely affect bone density.

Case Study

Betty is sixty-nine and has never been on estrogen replacement therapy. She gets into the shower one morning and reaches up to adjust the nozzle. She experiences a stubborn pain that persists for several weeks.

Finally, she tires of waiting for it to go away and makes an appointment with her doctor. An examination reveals that her spine is fractured in several places. Betty is baffled. She didn't fall or experience any other trauma, and over-the-counter pain medications seem to help well enough. The doctor prescribes a course of treatment including high calcium intake, as much exercise as she can realistically handle, and a review of her diet and medications. He explains to her that her best hope is to slow progression of the osteoporosis. Over time, the pain becomes more extreme and persistent. Gradually, Betty uses more and more painkillers and learns to live with the disease. She watches herself shrink and her back bend into the characteristic dowager's hump—a curve in the upper back causing the neck and head to hang forward. Betty hopes for the discovery of additional interventions or therapies for her condition.

Conclusion

Osteoporosis is not a disease with a single, targetable cause, like a viral infection. It is the result of prolonged bone loss due to many causes, some more significant for you than for others. To manage bone loss, you must understand the risk factors that apply specifically to you and act to minimize them. You cannot prevent osteoporosis just by listening to your body, because by the time you have symptoms, it is too late. Your body exhibits no signs of discomfort or pain as the calcium is spirited out of your bones and only tells you that something has gone wrong when you suffer a painful, irreversible fracture. Prevention is not complicated, but it requires foresight. Below is a handy table that lists the most common risk factors for osteoporosis. Use it to assess your risks and plan a personal prevention program.

Osteoporosis Risk Factors

AGING

Bones of all races and both genders become less sturdy with age

Age-related decreases in sex hormone levels cause bone loss in men and women

Secondary hyperparathyroidism, a disease of aging, causes bone loss

Age-related reduction in physical activity causes bone loss

Calcium absorption falls due to declining stomach acid levels

GENDER

Women

Women lose bone earlier than men

Age-related shrinkage of women's bones is more ruinous

Falling estrogen levels promote rapid bone loss

Menopausal women can lose as much as five to seven percent of bone mass per year, for three to five years

Men

Men suffer less because they do not live as long as women

The number of male osteoporosis cases is expected to rise with life expectancy

Osteoporosis tends to occur ten to fifteen years later than in women

Male bone breaks down less ruinously than female bone

Falling testosterone levels increase bone loss

Higher male levels of corticosteroids, growth hormones, circulating prolactin, and blood calcium increase bone loss

Men do not experience the massive bone loss characteristic of menopause

Testosterone stimulates bone and muscle growth

Falling levels of testosterone and estradiol contribute to male osteoporosis

Hypogonadal osteoporosis is treated with testosterone replacement therapy

BODY TYPE
Small skeletons carrying little weight lose bone quickly

Larger frames stimulate bone renewal

Thin people lose bone faster

ANCESTRY
Family
Premature or rapid bone loss may be hereditary

Genes linked to deficient vitamin D metabolism may increase bone loss

A gene that controls a type of bone-producing collagen may suffer hereditary mutation

Race
Caucasians, Asians, North American Inuit, and Hispanics are at greatest risk

African-Americans are at lowest risk

African-American women lose bone more slowly

African-Americans have denser vertebra

African Nantu women never suffer from calcium deficiency, seldom break a bone, and almost never lose a tooth

LIFESTYLE AND DIET
Physical Activity
Lack of weight-bearing stress leads to weak bones

Impact-loading and weight-bearing exercise stimulates bone formation

Bed-ridden patients lose bone rapidly

Tobacco and Caffeine
Smoking may accelerate bone loss (inconclusive)

Smoking may prompt earlier menopause, accelerating bone loss in women

Smokers weigh less (an additional risk factor)

Those with high caffeine intake have lower average bone mass

Alcohol
Alcohol abusers suffer greater bone loss

Alcoholics tend to eat poorly (an additional risk factor)

continued

Heavy alcohol use damages liver function and impedes vitamin D metabolism

Heavy drinking impairs osteoblast function

Heavy drinkers are excessively thin (an additional risk factor)

Diet
Low milk consumption during growth years leads to weaker skeletons

Excessive protein intake, particularly meat, depletes blood-calcium levels and releases calcium from bone

Low-fat diets are associated with a two-fold greater rate of bone loss

High levels of vitamin A may increase the risk of osteoporosis

Deficiency of vitamin K_2 impedes bone metabolism

Vitamin D deficiency in children weakens bones

Some lactose-intolerant individuals are unable to absorb dietary vitamin D

Excessive dietary phosphorous (too many soft drinks) decreases calcium absorption

Soft drinks often replace milk during the crucial teenage years

Pharmaceutical Drugs
Steroids
Thyroid hormone
GNRH analogs
LHRH-agonists
Anticonvulsants
Anticoagulants

3

Diagnosing Osteoporosis

How can you tell if you have osteoporosis? Sadly, the first step is often a patient's recognition of pain, after which a visit to the doctor leads to tests and a firm diagnosis. Unfortunately, if pain is already present it will almost inevitably have been caused by a fracture. Such fractures can be treated, but not reversed or healed. Osteoporosis is called a silent disease because it prepares the ground for massive damage without presenting any noticeable symptoms. The pain indicates that fracturing has begun and the bone has started losing its structure. The damage is irreversible. Although preventive measures may prevent further degeneration, the patient must get used to living with chronic pain.

To avoid this scenario, you should carefully study the risk factors described in chapter 2. They will help you consider whether you need to check your bone mineral density.

In particular, postmenopausal women have an important decision to make—to take or not to take hormone replacement therapy. Once all factors and treatment options have been weighed, the risk is often considered slight. Bone-mass measurements at this time will help you make an informed decision. They will also help track the effectiveness of the therapy and help your doctor maintain the correct dose.

Those using corticosteroid medications should be tested regularly to track possible accelerated bone loss. These lifesaving drugs and some others actually increase the rate of bone loss, especially when they are used for long periods. If you are such a patient, your doctor should be monitoring your bones at least once a year, if not more frequently.

If you have any reason to suspect that your bones are weakening, do not delay. Get a diagnosis. Osteoporosis is entirely preventable in most cases.

What Tests Can Show

Most of the tests described here are based on internal imaging, in most cases using X-ray technology. Metabolic tests and portable ultrasound measurement of bone-mineral density are convenient but not sufficiently reliable diagnostic tools. At best, they suggest possible bone loss and lead to more definitive testing. Bone imaging is the only way to obtain reliable information about bone loss.

To confirm absolutely that one is experiencing a particular rate of bone loss requires two or more tests separated by a significant period, usually one year. If you are afraid of thinning bones, will you have to wait a year to find out? The answer is no. A prognosis is made by comparing your results with the average bone density of others. Doctors can thus assess the likelihood of osteopenia (significant pre-osteoporotic bone loss without fractures), osteoporosis, and fractures.

Preliminary Testing

There is no substitute for bone-imaging technology in the diagnosis of osteoporosis. However, a doctor will often order bone scans only after noticing certain metabolic changes in the body. These changes can be detected in urine and blood, and tests may help identify the specific causes of an individual's bone loss. In testing these body fluids, laboratory workers are looking for markers—evidence of disease activity in the body. For example, certain concentrations of a specific protein—N-telopeptide—in the urine indicate heightened activity of osteoclasts and a probable ongoing decrease in bone density.

URINE TESTS

Urine can be tested for calcium levels and osteoclast activity.

Calcium Levels

Although massive bone loss would normally be accompanied by high levels of calcium in the urine, simply finding high calcium levels there is not a definitive diagnosis. Excessive urinary calcium may be caused by increased absorption of dietary calcium. Furthermore, normal levels are no guarantee that bone loss is not occurring.

High levels of urinary calcium suggest a variety of diseases, including Cushing's syndrome (an excess of corticosteroid hormones), idiopathic hypercalcinuria (unexplained high-calcium urine levels), milk-alkalai syndrome (high-calcium blood levels due to excessive intake of calcium-containing drugs and milk), osteolytic bone disease (dissolution of bone tissue), osteoporosis, primary hyperparathyroidism (overactivity of the parathyroid glands), renal tubular acidosis (kidney dysfunction leading to high acid levels in the blood), sarcoidosis (inflammation of tissues throughout the body), or vitamin D intoxication. Low calcium levels in the urine indicate possible hypoparathyroidism (underactivity of the parathyroid glands), malabsorption (inability to absorb nutrients), renal osteodystrophy (any bone disease of metabolic origin), or vitamin D deficiency. Although some of these disorders seem to increase urinary calcium output and some to slow it, one way or another most of them contribute directly to bone loss. The various causes of bone loss for a particular patient must be identified and prioritized. Only then can an appropriate therapy be devised.

Treatments aimed at decreasing bone resorption into the blood are normally expected to decrease calcium excretion, as are therapies that encourage bone formation. Testing during treatment may suggest the therapy's effectiveness but is not definitive. It is one of several diagnostic tools that must take the overall picture into account and require the interpretive skills of a practiced physician.

Osteoclast Activity (Bone Breakdown)

When osteoclast activity increases bone resorption, collagen breakdown increases. Collagen is the main protein found in bone and skin. Its breakdown produces the chemical hydroxyproline, which is passed into the urine. Hydroxyproline is considered a marker for the rate of bone turnover. Levels of this substance tend to double in post-menopausal women.

Another test identifies levels of a particular part of the collagen protein in bone, called the collagen cross-link, which passes unchanged from the bone into the urine. The rate at which cross-links are released into the urine is a measure of the rate at which osteoclasts are resorbing bone. This test is used to monitor bone cell activity and the patient's response to therapy.

BLOOD TESTS

Certain biochemical markers found in blood may help identify the disease(s) responsible for bone loss. The following types of measurement can be made from blood samples:

Calcium

In those with actively thinning bones, such as osteoporotic post-menopausal women, blood-calcium levels as well as urine-calcium levels may be normal even though calcium is being constantly removed from bones. In other words, normal blood-calcium levels offer no reassurance that you are not suffering bone loss. A small increase in blood calcium levels may suggest overall loss, but this is often offset by a corresponding decrease in calcium absorption that renders the increase invisible. High blood-calcium levels alone may indicate increased intestinal absorption of calcium (a good thing) or increased bone resorption of bone minerals into the blood (a bad thing).

Osteoblast Activity (Bone Formation)

Osteoblasts (bone-building cells) manufacture a protein called osteocalcin that is not actually used in bone but is released into the bloodstream as bone is formed. Measurement of this protein in the blood indicates the rate of bone formation. However, it does not eliminate the possibility that bone resorption by osteoclasts may be taking place at an even faster pace. For example, menopausal women exhibit elevated osteocalcin levels because bone formation is speeding up, even though bone resorption speeds up even more, and overall bone mineral density is falling.

Osteoblasts leave another telltale marker in the blood—alkaline phosphatase. Tests to monitor this enzyme have become an increasingly popular way to measure levels of bone-formation activity. Once again, the fact that bone is being formed by osteoblasts doesn't mean that overall bone loss is not taking place. However, when accompanied by low parathyroid hormone levels, osteoblast activity can mean that bone renewal is in a state of relative balance or positive growth.

Testing of blood and urine for markers of bone formation and resorption can be used to calculate the rate of bone loss over time and may help determine the urgency of avoiding specific risk factors. But the skeleton must also be examined to see if there is a risk of imminent fracture. Bone mineral density (BMD) is in most cases a good indicator of bone condition. Measuring it depends upon X-ray and other imaging technologies.

Bone Mineral Density

Although the density of most substances is usually measured in weight over volume, bone mineral density (BMD) is measured in grams per square inch. A variety of scientific instruments is used to assess the strength of bone by determining its permeability to various types of energy, such as ultrasound or X-rays. To be useful, the measurement must be very precise. Remember, bone is not a dense lump of matter but an airy latticework with considerable space distributed among the inner trabeculae. Bone density falls gradually, but there's nothing gradual about the osteoporotic change in shape and function of bones. They continue to work normally for years or decades until they fracture suddenly and traumatically. Whether to detect this tendency or to measure the effectiveness of treatment, changes in density must be measured over a period of time. To accurately identify a loss of 1 percent bone mass over a year, a significant amount, requires precise and reliable equipment.

To put your BMD measurement in context, it is compared against two standards. The first is the average bone mineral density of males or females with risk factors approximately similar to your own at the age (usually in their twenties) of their peak bone mass (T-score). The second is the average density for similar people of the same age (Z-score). The T-score shows how your current bone mineral density compares to what we assume was your own peak bone mass. The idea is to see how much your bone has changed. The Z-score comparison indicates how you are doing for your age, and whether you need more or less attention than others of your age with similar risk factors. Subsequent BMD measurements—usually a year or so later—are compared to your own previous score to determine your specific rate of bone loss, or gain if you have found an effective therapy.

WHICH BONES TO TEST

Accurate testing equipment has developed in recent decades to the point where the density of any part of the skeleton can be measured. The spine and the hip are often used as general indicators of bone condition since these are the sites most likely to suffer initial fractures. For several reasons, the spine is considered a less reliable source of information—especially in elderly patients. For example, the normal osteoarthritis of aging results in bone outgrowths along the vertebrae. Scans of the spine may reveal more total bone mass even though the density of the inner trabeculae may be falling. Vertebrae that are fractured and compressed may show increased density due to the compression. The possible sites of earlier surgery may also confuse measurements. Some doctors will order readings of both spine and hip, but this increases costs and is not usually considered necessary. Measurements of total hip BMD are frequently used with some reliability to predict the possibility of fractures in both hip and spine. In certain infrequent cases, measurement of both hip and spine are ordered, usually when the principal causes of bone loss are metabolically different. For example, patients with primary or secondary hyperparathyroidism usually suffer much greater loss at the hip than at the spine. This is because parathyroid hormone tends to deplete hard, cortical bone more quickly than inner trabecular bone, and the hip is composed more of cortical than trabecular bone.

However, identifying the danger of possible fractures is only one use of BMD readings. They are also used to measure the effectiveness of restorative therapies over time. Once again, the type of bone tested is important, especially in relation to the type of therapy. The spinal vertebrae have more inner, trabecular bone and trabecular bone is more metabolically active. In general, they respond more quickly when conditions are favorable for bone growth. Depending on whether these conditions are induced by increased calcium intake, hormone replacement therapy, or the removal of an important risk factor such as corticosteroid drugs, each type of bone may be affected differently.

BONE-DENSITY TESTING

All methods of bone-density testing use machines to reproduce visual images of the interior of the body. These machines range from low-cost, portable ultrasound devices to sophisticated and expensive quantitative computerized tomography scanners. A new type of imaging, called amorphous silicon filmless digital X-ray detection, seems to provide what every doctor wants—a fast, inexpensive, and sensitive way to measure small changes in bone mass. All methods are described below in detail. A handy "At a Glance" table follows on page 58.

Portable Ultrasound Testing

Apart from high-end laboratory ultrasound scanners, described below, a variety of inexpensive, portable ultrasound scanners is available today. The machines transmit sound waves through the bone and measure their changes as they emerge. These machines do not provide images, merely numbers that rate your BMD. They measure bone density in the wrist or, more commonly, the heel. Manufacturers claim that measurements at these sites can be used to extrapolate the condition of bone elsewhere in the body, but most doctors prefer to make further tests before forming a diagnosis. Nevertheless, these cursory measurements may identify the need for more thorough testing. The advantage of these machines is their portability, relatively low cost, and ease of use, since they do not require a licensed X-ray operator.

X-ray Imaging

Traditional X-ray imaging works by sending radiation through the body and capturing the emerging rays on photographic film. It shows the shape and general condition of the skeleton very clearly and will reveal fractures, but doesn't provide much inner detail and cannot be used to predict the danger of future breakage. High-density matter, such as bone, forms a whiter image on film, while low-density matter like air appears black. Other matter such as skin and soft tissue appears in various shades of gray. The visible resolution of the gray areas is poor, and bone depletion is only detectable on a scale of 30 percent or so. More subtle changes are undetectable. However, X-ray technology is used by other devices in new ways that are sufficiently sophisticated to record the detail doctors need to evaluate bone density.

Quantitative Ultrasound Testing

Quantitative ultrasound technology measures the speed at which sound travels through any part of the body—the faster its passage, the thinner the bone—and uses the information to construct an image. Ultrasound's ability to detect movement is well known by pregnant women, whose first glimpse of their baby is often an ultrasound image.

Ultrasound measurements seem to provide a unique type of information about bone mass. They are now considered as effective as most other currently available methods of predicting the risk of fracture. This technology provides a different but useful picture of what's happening on both the inside and the outside of bones. In the future, it may be used to separately detect thinning of cortical (outer) and trabecular (inner) bone. This is considered theoretically possible because the two types of bone seem to affect ultrasound waves—and the resulting measurements—in distinct ways. Ultrasound is particularly useful because of its potential to detect the different causes of bone loss that may affect cortical and trabecular bone at different rates.

Single-Photon Absorptiometry (SPA)

Single-photon absorptiometry was introduced in 1960. It was one of the first effective ways to measure bone density. A densitometer passes gamma rays through the bone, and the emerging rays are measured. A high value of gamma radiation indicates greater bone density; a lower value suggests low density. When first introduced, there were many parts of the body that could not be measured by the SPA. It could only measure bones not surrounded by large amounts of muscle and other tissue, such as the heel and wrist. Later, improvements in the technology made it possible to measure forearm bones. This is a convenient site because both types of bone can be tested. The lower end of the radius of the forearm contains a high proportion of trabecular bone, about 26 percent and bone in the middle of the forearm has a high proportion of cortical bone, about 70 percent.

DUAL-PHOTON ABSORPTIOMETRY (DPA)

Dual-photon absorptiometry is a technical advance over single-photon absorptiometry, enabling the testing of the spine, the hip, and indeed, any site in the body.

Use of this technology is on the wane today. In spite of its very low level of radiation, it was replaced by other methods that emit even less. Also, DPA and SPA were slow, taking at least twenty minutes just to measure the spine. The hip often took twice as long. While patients suffered no discomfort, this increased the cost of use.

While the initial measurement from single- and dual-photon absorptiometry is quite accurate as part of a diagnosis of osteoporosis and a predictor of possible fractures, it is of less use when trying to determine changes in BMD over time, or the progression of bone loss.

Dual-Energy X-ray Absorptiometry (DEXA, DXA)

DEXA eschews gamma rays for old-fashioned X-rays, and does everything a photon absorptiometer can do at about ten times the speed. In addition, results are very accurate. Changes in BMD of just 1 to 4 percent in a year can be detected. This has been the procedure of choice for almost two decades now and was the first reliable way to monitor the progress of patients after they had been diagnosed and were receiving therapy.

Quantitative Computed Tomography (QCT)

QCT is a type of CAT (Computed Tomography) scan for bone which accurately measures BMD in the spine or elsewhere. A CT scanner is a large, doughnut-shaped scanner that rotates around the patient. Its great advantage is the ability to take measurements at the very center of spinal vertebrae. Its disadvantages include the patient's exposure to more radiation than the other methods described here. These are not dangerous levels by any means, but in general, less radiation is better.

Magnetic Resonance Imaging (MRI)

An MRI scanner is a large cylinder surrounded by a powerful electromagnet. The patient lies snugly within the cylinder while the magnetic field causes hydrogen atoms in the body to give off radio-frequency waves. These are measured and translated into a visual image on a computer screen. MRI is extremely accurate and flexible—it can create an image of bone slices at previously unobtainable angles, providing more clarity and detail than any other imaging technique. It may be used to examine bone at specific sites of fracture or disease, but it is not generally used to determine BMD. MRI scanners are known for their extremely noisy, claustrophobic test environment and have been known to trigger panic attacks in nervous patients.

Amorphous Silicon Filmless Digital X-ray Detection

Amorphous silicon filmless digital X-ray detection starts out like most other X-ray technologies but goes further. It does not require film to show results and provides excellent resolution. As esoteric as it sounds, amorphous silicon is ubiquitous today. Found in the flat-panel displays of many computers, especially laptops, its use as a detection technology provides great economy. It replaces X-ray film and significantly reduces the patient's exposure to X-rays. It displays high-resolution graphical results immediately on a computer screen. There is no waiting for film to develop. Best of all, this machine detects both osteoporosis and osteoarthritis at the same time. It provides convenient and accurate detection and is inexpensive enough to be found in the private offices of general practitioners.

READING BMD MEASUREMENTS

In looking at BMD test results, physicians are attempting to define a fracture threshold—an indication of how close one is to the risk of osteoporotic fracture. The calculation of this threshold takes into account several factors, including the bones tested, the patient's age and gender, and other risk factors.

The T-score (average peak BMD of similar-risk individuals) is measured as follows: a score of −1.0 indicates BMD 10 percent below the average for young adults; a score of −2.5 indicates a 25 percent discrepancy, and is usually the level at which people experience hip fractures. The National Osteoporosis Foundation of the United States, the World Health Organization, and The European Foundation for Osteoporosis have agreed upon standards for four general diagnostic categories of bone condition as measured by T-score. They are:

1. Normal—a score of −1.0 or more shows that BMD is within 10 percent of normal for young adults.

Bone Density Testing Methods at a Glance

Portable Ultrasound Testing
Not accurate, but may indicate the need for further testing.

X-ray Imaging
Better than nothing when other technology is unavailable, but does not provide great detail.

Quantitative Ultrasound Testing
Inexpensive, convenient, and fast, but not very reliable.

Single-Photon Absorptiometry (SPA)
Relatively reliable 1960s technology, able to identify advanced low density of certain bones, but not sufficiently refined to measure changes in bone mass year by year.

Dual-Photon Absorptiometry (DPA)
More flexible than SPA, and able to measure any part of the skeleton, but extremely slow and therefore expensive to operate.

Dual-Energy X-ray Absorptiometry (DEXA, DXA)
Accurate and fast, able to measure gradual changes in bone mass over periods of approximately one year.

Quantitative Computed Tomography (QCT)
Accurately measures bone mass of any part of any part of the skeleton.

Magnetic Resonance Imaging (MRI)
Extremely accurate, flexible, and intimidating technology. MRI scanners have been known for their extremely noisy, claustrophobic test environment, although newer machines are less traumatic.

Amorphous Silicon Filmless Digital X-ray Detection
Convenient, fast, and inexpensive.

2. Osteopenia—a T-score value from –1.0 to –2.5 indicates the approach of critical BMD levels.
3. Osteoporosis—T-score values below –2.5 predict immediate danger of bone collapse or fracture.
4. Severe osteoporosis—this term describes patients with T-scores below –2.5 who also have one or more osteoporotic fractures.

Notice that the third category—osteoporosis—is said to *predict* possible fractures. There is no certainty in this prediction. Even though two people may have similar T-scores, the way in which their bones have thinned (the quality of remaining bone) may leave one patient with more structural integrity than the other, and with a little more resistance to fractures.

Once bone loss has been diagnosed, you must keep track of further changes. These changes may be continued bone loss or—with appropriate therapy such as triple-A calcium supplementation (see chapter 5) and changed lifestyle habits such as regular weight-bearing exercise (see chapter 6)—increasing bone mineral density. You will also want to know, of course, if there is no change. In other words, periodic BMD measurements are essential. The possible frequency of these tests is limited by the sensitivity of the equipment. No machine can detect changes from one day to the next, but over the course of a year or two the changes—or the lack of change—are significant. Annual testing normally provides a clear indication of how you are doing. In future, more sensitive BMD measurements may be able to predict smaller changes over shorter periods. This may help reassure those at greatest risk that the measures being taken are working, but all therapy must be monitored over time. The problem evolves over several decades and repair takes years at best.

Conclusion

Given the variety of causes of bone loss and the fluctuations in the rate of loss due to age and other risk factors, and because severe bone loss can go on for years without the slightest noticeable symptom, bone testing is sooner or later essential for everyone. Cursory testing of blood, urine, and peripheral bone by portable ultrasound scanners can suggest the urgency of further testing by more accurate imaging machines. These provide a relative measure of your skeletal health and are also used to monitor subsequent developments and/or restorative therapies. Periodic testing for anyone with significant risk factors is essential. Depending on your particular risk factors, your doctor should schedule regular BMD tests with other routine tests, especially for women undergoing menopause and men entering old age. Men with high risk factors might consider BMD testing as early as age fifty. See the table on page 44 to quickly assess your risk factors.

4

Conventional
Therapies

Just as there are many identified (and probably still unidentified) causes of bone loss leading to osteopenia and osteoporosis, there are many ways to fight it. Lifestyle, exercise, diet, and medical treatment all play a part. This chapter discusses solutions normally termed "conventional" because they are in general and conventional use by most doctors and hospitals. It outlines the options likely to be considered by your M.D. Still, the classifications of conventional and alternative frequently overlap, so your doctor may be sympathetic to some of the therapies described in the next chapter on alternative therapies.

Successful alternative therapies often become conventional, such as the wide use of St. John's wort in Germany by many general practitioners. There is talk of alternative versus traditional medicine and natural versus pharmaceutical treatments, but these are not useful debates. You should at all costs avoid choosing therapies based on whether they fall into the category of "conventional" or of "alternative" medicine and simply seek out those that work for you. Don't forget, your doctor is your primary health-care consultant in this process of self-learning.

. . .

Anything that increases bone mass is a potential therapy against osteoporosis, but the efficacy of a particular approach depends upon your own particular causes of bone loss. Everyone loses bone with age, but while a particular risk factor such as poor diet may be a significant factor for one person, it could be relatively insignificant for someone else. This chapter will help you design a personal prevention and treatment program.

Estrogen Replacement Therapy

For decades, estrogen replacement therapy (ERT) was considered the only preventive measure for osteoporosis. Unfortunately, it was only available for women, some of whom were soon excluded as the risk of uterine cancer became known. Still estrogen may play a role in the prevention of bone loss in men. Of all risk factors, the postmenopausal avalanche of bone loss experienced by almost all women is the most dramatic. It outweighs most other risk factors except for severe illness like poliomyletis or perhaps the accumulated effects of long-term corticosteroid therapy. Addressing other factors such as lifestyle and exercise may help to slow bone loss, but the effectiveness of this approach varies from one individual to another.

Lifestyle changes made in youth or early adulthood may help you reach peak bone mass at a later age, giving you more bone to lose before complications set in, but menopause will still make significant inroads into your skeletal stores of calcium. Under no circumstances should any woman ignore the importance of preventive measures before, during, and after menopause. Still, even those who do not begin ERT promptly—as long as they begin within a few years of menopause—can still benefit.

Estrogen production virtually stops with natural menopause, at which point the rate of bone turnover speeds up significantly. Osteoblasts begin to create new bone at an unprecedented rate, but the osteoclasts are even more aggressive and the overall result is a continuous net drain of calcium from bone.

For estrogen replacement therapy to prevent or slow this metabolic change, it must be maintained throughout the normal period of menopause. When therapy is discontinued and bone loss picks up again, it is not at the accelerated postmenopausal pace. It is generally closer to the more moderate rate of loss taking place when therapy began. There are, therefore, two advantages to hormone replacement therapy: First, it diminishes bone loss and maintains a stronger skeleton. Second, it alleviates many other common, unpleasant effects of menopause.

Therapy is usually begun at menopause and maintained for seven to ten years. Studies have shown that hormone replacement reduces the risk of osteoporotic fractures of the hip and forearm by about one-third, and fractures of the spine by more than a half. Hormone replacement therapy is not a cure for osteoporosis, nor will it completely arrest bone loss. But if it is taken for this period, it removes a potent risk factor that otherwise leads most women down a dangerous path of bone loss and a toward a prognosis of early osteoporosis.

The ideal time to begin hormone replacement is when the ovaries stop working and your natural supplies of estrogen begin to dwindle. Overall bone loss begins at menopause but is slowed dramatically by the use of estrogen drugs. The sooner you take it, the less bone you'll lose. It can even be taken up a year or two after the onset of menopause, although some bone loss has already taken place and a late start is not recommended. Remember, estrogen therapy prevents or slows bone loss but does not rebuild bone already lost.

In earlier times, osteoporosis was but one of many signs of age-related degeneration. However, global life expectancy has risen dramatically since 1950 to its present sixty-six years, so most women worldwide live long beyond menopause. In highly industrialized countries many women reach menopause with more than one-third of their lives yet to be lived. Consider also that 55 percent of people over sixty and 65 percent of eighty-year-olds are women, and that by 2050 one-fifth of the world's population will be over sixty. Osteoporosis often makes those years difficult and painful, and the cost to society (see chapter 7) is increasing dramatically as people live longer. However, it can be easily prevented in most cases.

Estrogen for Men

Estrogen is said to be a female hormone because it is responsible for certain feminine characteristics and functions in the body. Some of these functions exist in men as well, just as testosterone provides certain necessary male characteristics in women, such as sex drive. Estrogen therapy has been tested in men with mixed results. A study at Hartford Hospital in Connecticut was designed to measure the effects of estrogen on bone turnover in men. The researchers also measured its effects on the cardiovascular system. High doses of estrogen are known to lead to cholesterol problems, but very low doses lessen these dangers to the heart and actually raise HDL (good) cholesterol levels in men, just as they do in women. Estrogen therapy also decreased levels of fibrinogen, an agent that increases the danger of blood clots. Some men suffered breast tenderness and heartburn, but none suffered reduced libido. Estrogen inhibits the action of osteoclasts in men as it does in women and can be helpful, although the side effects mentioned above might cause some men to avoid it.

WHY TAKE HORMONE REPLACEMENT THERAPY?

Estrogen acts directly on the intestine to increase calcium absorption. It also stimulates the synthesis of vitamin D in the kidneys, which enhances absorption even more, reducing bone loss. But this is only one advantage of estrogen replacement. For many women it effectively controls some of the most common and unpleasant features of menopause, including hot flashes, sleep disturbances, stress, incontinence, urinary tract infections, vaginal dryness, skin wrinkling and inelasticity, low energy levels, lessened sex drive, depression, and mood swings. There is evidence that it may prevent or delay the development of dementia and Alzheimer's disease in older women. Most significant of all is its effect on the risk of heart disease. With correct dosage, it effectively counters abnormal and harmful buildup of bad (HDL) cholesterol and maintains healthy levels of fibrinogen (a blood-clotting agent), thus reducing the risk of heart disease and stroke. It is no surprise than many women are happy to embark on a regimen of hormone replacement therapy. Nevertheless, you should be aware of these important risks.

RISKS OF HORMONE REPLACEMENT

Despite its many benefits, hormone replacement therapy is not a magic bullet. Most doctors are cautious about tampering with any aspect of the endocrine (hormonal) system, not just the female sex hormones. Introducing the right amount of hormones at the right time is not easy. Dozens of these chemical messengers interact in complex ways, sometimes producing unanticipated results. The key to good hormone replacement therapy is to maintain correct hormonal balance by testing and adjusting the dosage for each individual. Doctors must carefully weigh the pros and cons of HRT before prescribing it, and when they do you should expect a clear explanation of the immediate and long-term risks for your particular case. You should also expect regular follow-up examinations to find and maintain the best dosing schedule for you.

Cancer of the Uterus

The most serious threat of estrogen replacement therapy (ERT) is endometrial hyperplasia (overgrowth of the lining of the uterus) which often leads to endometrial cancer, especially after long-term use of estrogen (more than ten years). ERT became very popular for the first time in the 1960s, providing a very large population base for statistical analysis. A decade later it had become clear that women receiving estrogen alone had a significantly increased risk of developing endometrial cancer. Fortunately, the addition of progesterone (the other female hormone) or progestin (synthetic progesterone) significantly reduces this risk (see below), although its effect on bone loss is negligible. This combination, nowadays widely used, is referred to as Hormone Replacement Therapy (HRT).

A major clinical trial started in 1987 and called PEPI (postmenopausal estrogen/progestin interventions trial) showed that the risk of serious endometrial overgrowth is unacceptably high in women taking estrogen replacement alone, except for those whose uteruses had been removed by hysterectomy. Nowadays, these women are given combination therapy, and the risk of hyperplasia (overgrowth of the cells lining the uterus) and cancer is significantly reduced. However, progesterone or progestin is not given to women with thrombophlebitis (blood clots in the legs) or liver disease since it can worsen these conditions.

Breast Cancer

A significant number of women will not even consider hormone replacement therapy because they fear breast cancer. Most of them believe the risk is an established fact and never even consult their doctors. However, while some health professionals believe that the link between HRT and breast cancer is clear, others are still waiting to see more evidence. If you have a history of breast cancer in your family, you should speak to your doctor, and know that whatever his/her opinion, it may not be shared by all other doctors. Some studies have shown up to a 30 or even 50 percent increase in the incidence of breast cancer for women on long-term ERT (ten years or more), but others have found no increase at all. It remains a highly controversial topic.

Other Risks

Hormone replacement therapy is used cautiously on women with uncontrolled high blood pressure, migraines, former or existing blood clots in the leg or lung, diabetes, preexisting gallstones, mild liver disease, endometriosis, and uterine fibroids (benign tumors in the uterus). These complications are listed on many HRT medications as contraindications—factors in a patient's condition that may make it unwise to pursue therapy. HRT does not cause these problems, but if they already exist, it may make them worse. However, these contraindications were formulated in earlier times, when suggested dosage was much higher than is common today. If any of them apply to you, you should not expect to be necessarily excluded from therapy, but you should expect to be carefully monitored.

HRT is often denied to women with a history of abnormal vaginal bleeding or severe liver disease. There is also fear that patients with a history of melanoma (skin cancer) may be susceptible to recurrences when taking hormone replacement. And some doctors who prefer to err on the side of caution will deny HRT to women with a personal or family history of breast cancer. There are, however, other therapies that use hormonelike drugs with less risk than estrogen (see below).

Before making a decision to pursue hormone replacement therapy, it is important to balance the above risks against the risks of osteoporosis and heart disease. This evaluation should be based primarily on your personal history, family history, blood pressure, and cholesterol values. Weigh everything carefully and use your doctor as a professional consultant to make an informed decision.

PROGESTERONE AND PROGESTIN

Progesterone, after estrogen, is the second female hormone produced by the ovaries. It has no noticeable role in preventing bone loss, but its replacement in HRT is used to diminish the risk of endometrial cancer. Its role in menstruating women is to facilitate pregnancy by causing the endometrium (lining of the uterus) to thicken in preparation for the implantation of a fertilized egg. If pregnancy does not occur, progesterone and estrogen secretion both stop and the lining is shed along with the unfertilized egg (menstruation).

Normally, the menstrual period ceases after menopause. However, when progesterone (or a synthetic formulation called progestin) is added as a complement to the estrogen in hormone replacement therapy, the monthly period will continue. Progesterone prevents the overgrowth (hyperplasia) of cells that is encouraged by estrogen therapy alone and reduces the risk of cancer. Progestins are sometimes even used to treat cancer. Also, the addition of progestin to HRT enables doctors to use a lower estrogen dosage, which reduces the overall risk even more. This combination is also known as combination therapy or PERT (progestin/estrogen replacement therapy).

Progesterone may be a natural hormone, but when taken by mouth it is rapidly broken down in the liver before it has a chance to get into the bloodstream. In other words, it is poorly absorbed. Progestin—a synthetic, absorbable alternative with similar metabolic effects—was designed for easy use. It is available under several brand names from a variety of pharmaceutical manufacturers. However, progestin also diminishes (but does not entirely eliminate) estrogen's tendency to elevate HDL (good) cholesterol levels and protect the cardiovascular system. Natural progesterone does not diminish the advantages of estrogen in this way, so efforts have been made to prepare a formulation of the natural hormone that will make it more usable. A more absorbable form called micronized progesterone is now available, and others will presumably follow.

Progesterone and progestin are used not only for postmenopausal hormone replacement but also to treat abnormal uterine bleeding and as a component of birth-control pills. They have also been used in an attempt to treat premenstrual syndrome. This application may be highly marketable, but it has little scientific support and has caused considerable controversy.

Women who have had a hysterectomy (removal of the uterus, and sometimes also the ovaries and fallopian tubes) are not given progesterone replacement. Since they no longer have a uterus, there is no risk of endometrial cancer. They do not need progestin and benefit from estrogen alone without increased risk.

TESTOSTERONE

In addition to estrogen and progesterone, your doctor may prescribe supplementation of testosterone. Testosterone (an androgen, or male hormone) is produced in the ovaries and adrenal glands. When the ovaries shut down at menopause, they stop producing testosterone. The adrenal secretions continue but do not produce enough testosterone to keep up premenopausal levels. A postmenopausal woman's supply of the male hormone is therefore often in short supply, with several consequences—one of which is impaired bone regrowth.

Although estrogen usually prevents bone loss—or at least profound bone loss—by inhibiting the activity of osteoclasts, there is evidence that testosterone supplementation complements it by stimulating osteoblasts that actually rebuild bone. Testosterone is also given to women who have not obtained satisfactory relief from menopausal hot flashes or who are complaining of low libido.

DOSAGE

As with most types of hormone therapy, dosage and scheduling of estrogen and progesterone or progestin is a tricky affair. Normally in premenopausal women progesterone secretion occurs only in the second half of the menstrual cycle while estrogen is secreted continuously, except during the period of bleeding. Progesterone thickens the lining of the uterus in preparation for the implantation of a fertilized egg. If no fertilization occurs, both progesterone and estrogen levels fall and the endometrium is shed along with the unfertilized egg during the monthly period. In postmenopausal women—depending on the dosing schedule—HRT can have the same function, sometimes producing periodlike activity and discomfort, even though there is no egg to be shed. This side effect unfortunately causes some women to discontinue hormone replacement therapy, but there are some dosing schedules that bring an end to monthly bleeding.

There are several ways of combining hormone drugs. As long as they have not undergone a hysterectomy, women on estrogen therapy usually also receive progesterone replacement. This takes the form of either progestin or an absorbable progesterone. Its usefulness depends upon the extent to which estrogen therapy encourages overgrowth of a woman's uterine lining. For some, the threat is minimal and they take this hormone for just a few days every few months. Others may take a little each day, along with estrogen. Some take it for ten days a month. There are rules of thumb, but each woman tends to have different needs and to react uniquely to her dosing schedule. The degree of hyperplasia (overgrowth of the cells lining the uterus, raising the possibility of cancer) varies from woman to woman and is the entire focus of progesterone replacement. If hyperplasia is pronounced, you will need to take progesterone for a longer period each month to ensure that the endometrial lining is completely shed.

There are two general ways in which progesterone or progestin is combined with estrogen. One is a continuous combination, using both daily. This prevents the monthly thickening and shedding of the endometrium and generally causes monthly bleeding to come to a halt within about a year, if not sooner. For obvious reasons it is relatively popular among women, but your doctor may not be satisfied that the threat of endometrial hyperplasia is sufficiently diminished.

The alternative is sequential dosing—closer to the normal cycle of hormonal secretion for premenopausal women. Women take estrogen alone for two weeks, then estrogen with progestin or absorbable progesterone for two weeks. This therapy provokes a menstrual-like cycle, eliminating the endometrium during a predictable period of bleeding.

A variation on the second method is a so-called cyclic dosing schedule, similar to contraceptive dosing—three weeks on, one week off with progesterone replacement only in the second half of the dosing period. This mimics even more closely the hormonal cycles of the menstrual period. It is not unusual for women on this regimen to complain of bloating and other familiar symptoms of premenstrual syndrome (PMS). They may also experience headaches, sore breasts, moodiness and acne. Changing the type of progestin or progesterone sometimes helps.

On the other hand, if you have a history of recurrent endometrial cancer, your doctor may be reluctant to put you on any sort of estrogen replacement therapy, in which case progestin or progesterone is unnecessary. Don't worry: There are other ways to maintain your bone mineral density. The important thing is to be aware of the threat of menopause and to act accordingly. Don't assume, because you are otherwise in good health, that you are not at risk. After all, when it comes to bone loss, there is no discomfort and there are no symptoms. But there are consequences.

The choice of regimen is not arbitrary. It must be tailor-made for you. Your doctor should be able to explain exactly why your particular prescription is appropriate.

Delivery

The most common form of hormone replacement medications come in pill form, but skin patches are also available, similar in mechanism to nicotine patches. They are convenient and inexpensive and need to be replaced only every few days. Pills are generally taken daily.

Estrogen promotes some different metabolic effects depending on the way it is delivered. After estrogen from a pill is released into the bloodstream, it passes through the liver *en masse* before entering general circulation. Estrogen delivered from a transdermal patch enters the general circulation first and passes through the liver a little at a time. This may be significant for those with cholesterol problems, because high estrogen levels in the liver promote a general reduction in circulating cholesterol and an elevation of HDL (good) cholesterol. The patch also raises HDL levels, but not as significantly as oral estrogen. If you have cholesterol problems, your doctor may take this into account. However, the greater portion of estrogen's ability to reduce the threat of heart disease may be its direct effect on blood vessels rather than on cholesterol levels. If so, the means of delivery is less significant. As for its effect on bone metabolism, there is no known difference between the effects of orally delivered and transdermally delivered estrogen.

Since cigarette smoke is toxic, it passes quickly into the liver. There, it reacts with estrogen to reduce its effectiveness. Since transdermal estrogen patches deliver the estrogen into general circulation first and avoid this concentration in the liver, they may be more effective for smokers.

There are also some concerns that estrogen that circulates via the liver may cause or exacerbate gallstones and high blood pressure. This theory is so far unsubstantiated and quite theoretical. Your doctor is unlikely to take it into account unless you are particularly susceptible to or are currently suffering from either of these complaints.

Estrogen creams are also available for topical (local) applications, usually to treat vaginal dryness or atrophic vaginitis (poor or insufficient vaginal lining). As you might imagine, such creams provide no significant benefit to your bones. If this is the only estrogen therapy you use, progesterone replacement is unnecessary.

Types of Estrogen and Progesterone Drugs

To avoid unnecessary confusion, we have spoken of estrogen and progestin drugs as if they were unique. In reality, there is a variety of available estrogens and progestins. They go under generic chemical names and many trademarks. The most common estrogens are beta estradiol and its derivatives—estrone, estriol, and conjugated estrogens. Progesterone is replaced by any of these progestins—medroxyprogesterone acetate, norethindrone acetate, mesgesterol acetate, or norgestrel—or by natural progesterone.

Some questions about hormone replacement remain to be answered. Exactly when is the best time to begin HRT—as menopause approaches or only after ovulation has come to a permanent end? How long should it continue—five years at least, but is ten better, or even twelve? To what extent does estrogen's tendency to elevate HDL (good cholesterol) levels actually prevent heart attacks and stroke? How much estrogen is just right? How little is effective? And, of course, can a clear link be established between estrogen replacement therapy and breast cancer? Ask your doctor. He or she should be aware of the latest developments.

Alternatives to Hormones

A variety of nonhormonal drugs has been developed and is under development to counter the negative effects of estrogen loss. Some of them are just as potent in preventing bone loss.

SELECTIVE ESTROGEN
RECEPTOR MODULATORS (SERMS)

Selective estrogen receptor modulators (SERMs) act like hormones but pose less risk.

Tamoxifen

Tamoxifen, a nonhormonal compound, provides some of the properties of estrogen without its disadvantages. It is often prescribed for women with a particular susceptibility to breast cancer or osteoporosis. It seems to act as an anti-estrogen in breast tissue but like estrogen in other parts of the body. Breast tumors have a protein on their surface that acts as a receptor for estrogen. Tamoxifen binds with this receptor and inhibits tumor activity. Some studies in postoperative breast cancer survivors taking tamoxifen have shown success in treating and preventing recurrence and growth of new tumors.

Tamoxifen's estrogenlike activity is also weaker in the uterus. Like estrogen it may promote hyperplasia (overgrowth) of uterine lining cells in some women, but it seems to pose less risk. Nevertheless, women taking tamoxifen should be carefully monitored.

Like estrogen, tamoxifen elevates HDL (good) cholesterol and lowers LDL (bad) cholesterol levels. It has been shown to measurably reduce bone loss in the hip and spine.

Raloxifene

Raloxifene has been linked with reduced risk of breast cancer and heart disease in postmenopausal women, so it has effects similar to those of estrogen, although it does not deal with these risks quite as effectively as estrogen. Still, its positive effects on blood levels of triglycerides, the fat-transporters Apo-A and Apo-B, and fibrinogen, the blood-clotting agent, surpass those of estrogen, and it seems to carry an even lower risk of breast cancer than tamoxifen.

. . .

Other compounds have been developed by the pharmaceutical industry to act in similar ways—to promote estrogenlike activity in the cardio-vascular system and bones—where it is beneficial, and antiestrogenic effects where is might be harmful—such as in breast tissue. Droloxifene and idoxifene are two such drugs. If you cannot or do not want to take estrogen therapy, ask your doctor about these alternatives.

Calcitonin

Calcitonin is a hormone made in the thyroid gland alongside thyroid hormone. It is named after calcium because its main role is calcium management. It affects bone by diminishing the activity of osteoclasts and thus reducing bone resorption. It is therefore protective of bone in a way similar to estrogen, but it can do more. The higher your rate of bone turnover, the more dramatic the effects of calcitonin. Even fifteen to twenty years after menopause, women with existing osteoporotic fractures can benefit from this hormone, gaining bone mass and developing fewer or no new fractures. Calcitonin derived from various animal sources, especially salmon, is widely used today.

Calcitonin can be applied through a subcutaneous (under the skin) injection or as a nasal spray. Like estrogen replacement, calcitonin only provides protection when taken continuously. As therapy begins, it may provoke nausea and mild discomfort in the digestive system, but these side effects tend to diminish in time. Itching can also occur around the site of an injection, but this too usually disappears. If not, it can generally be preempted by a mild antihistamine taken a half hour or so before the injection. However, the nasal application avoids these side effects and is more convenient.

Calcitonin has one additional benefit—it seems to relieve pain. This was a welcome but surprising discovery for researchers who are still trying to identify its painkilling mechanism. It has been suggested that calcitonin may stimulate production of endorphins, the body's own natural painkillers. Also, its direct effect upon osteoclasts (cells that break down bone) may have something to do with it. Combined with its ability to rebuild even severely diminished bone mass, this makes calcitonin very attractive to patients with existing osteoporosis. People with vertebral fractures often suffer severe back pain. This pain was formerly treated with codeine or other morphine-derived pain medications, but these drugs often provoke constipation and hard bowel movements, causing back strain and further pain. Calcitonin has no such side effect.

Calcitonin has been approved by the U.S. Food and Drug Administration for the treatment of postmenopausal osteoporosis, although not for its prevention. Nevertheless, it is often prescribed to newly menopausal women who are in danger of bone loss and for whom estrogen or combination therapy poses too great a risk or fear.

Bisphosphonates

Bisphosphonates (also called diphosphonates) are a family of compounds with an irresistible attraction to calcium. Once introduced into the body, bisphosphonates head straight for the bones and attach themselves to the outer surface, especially at the sites of bone turnover where osteoclasts are trying to get to work. (Remember that bone is naturally broken down and rebuilt in isolated patches—see chapter 1.) Bisphosphonates bind to the bone and have a chemical structure that is hard for osteoclasts (bone resorption cells) to break down. Also, the chemical structure of this layer somehow inhibits replication of osteoclasts, diminishing their effectiveness and slowing bone resorption even more. You can imagine them as forming a sort of protective laminate that gradually covers the bone surface.

Early bisphosphonates were not entirely trustworthy, but newer members of this family provide an alternative for women who cannot or will not take estrogen. However, although a good way to prevent bone loss, bisphosphonates do not provide the same additional benefits as estrogen or SERMs.

ETIDRONATE

The first commercially available bisphosphonate was etidronate (all bisphosphonates end in "–dronate"). It is used rarely today. Its usefulness was somewhat tempered by suspicions that continuous use caused structural abnormalities in bone, and it was therefore used only intermittently— for just two weeks out of twelve or as a fifteen-week regimen. Nevertheless, tests with etidronate were promising enough to encourage clinical trials and the search for less objectionable bisphosphonates. This led to the development of alendronate—the first bisphosphonate to be approved by the FDA for the treatment of osteoporosis.

ALENDRONATE

Alendronate is a more potent protector of bone mass and is simultaneously much less likely to cause structural abnormalities. Unlike etidronate, alendronate may be used daily for years. The potential side effects of the entire family of bisphosphonates tend to be gastrointestinal, but for alendronate they are slight—mild, infrequent cases of nausea, diarrhea and/or constipation. Dosage is just one pill per day, but taking it is a rather less than straightforward affair. Alendronate must be taken in the morning on a empty stomach with a full glass of water, at least thirty minutes before eating or drinking. Coffee or juice taken with the medication or too close to it will interfere with absorption, and you will not benefit from your dose. Also, you must not lie down again after taking it, since irritation of the esophagus (passage from the mouth to the stomach) may occur, sometimes severe enough to provoke ulcers. So it is important to remain upright.

Alendronate has been approved for the prevention of osteoporosis and appears to be as effective as estrogen in preventing bone loss, but, again, does not afford the other benefits of estrogen.

A study carried out at the Oregon Health Sciences University showed that alendronate was successful in improving BMD at several sites in the male skeleton. This is the first treatment that has been specifically tested on men, and it is hoped that further studies will lead to FDA approval of a treatment for osteoporosis in males.

Residronate and Ibandronate

These are newer members of the bisphosphonate family that promote similar benefits while causing fewer gastrointestinal problems. Residronate was studied in Denmark in 1998 on a group of 111 postmenopausal women. After two years of treatment, women on this bisphosphonate had actually grown new bone. Even after therapy was discontinued, this group maintained better BMD values in the spine than a control group of women not on residronate.

Residronate may be ideal for patients with osteoporosis—in other words, those with dangerously low BMD and existing fractures. It takes decades for bones to reach the point of fracture, but once the first one has occurred, others tend to follow quite rapidly. To avoid this domino effect, fast-acting therapies are needed to strengthen the skeleton quickly and maintain the structural integrity of as-yet undamaged bones. Residronate is one such candidate. Recent studies in North America, Europe, and Australia followed the progress of almost four thousand postmenopausal women with osteoporosis taking residronate. After just one year the risk of new vertebral fractures was reduced by over 60 percent. Side effects included back pain and joint pain, but gastrointestinal complaints seem to be extremely few—as long as it is taken on an empty stomach with water and one remains standing or sitting for a half-hour.

Calcium

Calcium is a common, naturally occurring mineral found in plants, animals, and rocks. It is not really a pharmaceutical product, although there are many pharmaceutical calcium preparations with significant differences. Still, it is the most conventional of all preventive osteoporosis therapies, although its use by itself may not be enough. Whether you are just trying to avoid the distant possibility of bone loss or you are suffering from advanced osteoporosis, your doctor will almost certainly suggest you increase your calcium intake. No matter what sort of hormone or nonhormone therapy you use to counter bone loss, calcium should be a part of it.

Calcium also has important benefits for the body above and beyond the protection of bone. It circulates continuously in small quantities in the blood, where its effects on the function of nerves (especially in the brain) and muscle (especially the heart) are critically important. Without adequate levels of serum calcium (calcium dissolved in blood) our hearts would stop beating and the brain's ability to send and receive messages along neural pathways would simply stop. Believe it or not, without calcium we would quickly die.

Luckily, our blood never runs out of calcium because we have a literally inexhaustible storehouse in our bones. There will always be enough calcium to keep the heart and brain going, but there may not always be enough to maintain the skeleton, which—as we know only too well—can suffer crippling structural breakdown.

We have known for a long time that bones need calcium—especially growing bones. The amount of calcium in the diet of children determines the future life span and health of their skeleton and cannot be overemphasized. On the other hand, calcium is not so hard to find. There is plenty in dairy products like milk, yogurt, ice cream, and cheese—even when low in fat—fish with bones, beans, greens (especially kale and broccoli), oranges, and dozens of other common foods. Still, we can use a lot more than we usually find in our food—a gram or two (1,000–2,000 mg) a day is recommended quite routinely for adults—and supplementation is never a bad idea, although the dietary portion of your calcium intake is generally the most absorbable. It is difficult to consume too much calcium. The only known side effect is constipation, although in large doses it may inhibit metabolism of the trace element zinc. Hypercalcemia (too much calcium in the blood) may result from the intake of too much vitamin D—which can disturb calcium balance in the body—or hyperparathyroidism (too much parathyroid hormone in the blood) rather than too much dietary calcium. If your calcium is fortified with vitamin D, make sure you don't take too much. If you are concerned about your vitamin D intake, consult your health care practitioner.

Calcium is best taken with meals. You may want to take it with fibrous foods to avoid constipation, but this will also prevent good absorption. The large quantities of calcium in spinach, for example, for the most part pass directly into the stool. Drinking lots of water throughout the day should help you maximize absorption and reduce constipation.

Calcium is an important component of the adult diet. There is never a time when we do not need calcium, but the amount we need to consume increases as we age. It's not that we need more calcium in the body—on the contrary, we just need to keep calcium levels constant. The trouble is, as we age our intestines become less effective. We absorb less and less calcium and need to eat more and more. Calcium is not particularly soluble in the first place, and what gets into our blood gets there by being dissolved. Even at the best of times we absorb barely one-third of what we eat. Older people also spend less time out in the sun, so vitamin D levels fall (sunshine stimulates vitamin D synthesis) and the kidneys work less effectively. As a result, more and more of the calcium we eat goes straight from the gastrointestinal tract into the urine. Even before reaching old age we absorb barely one-fifth of all the calcium we eat. This figure falls even more as the years go by, and each fall must be compensated for by greater and greater increases in dietary calcium and—even more important—by our ability to absorb it. For this reason, some increasingly soluble forms of calcium are beginning to appear on pharmacy shelves. To test the solubility of a calcium supplement, place it in white vinegar. It should dissolve within 30 minutes.

Increased calcium intake at any age is well known to slow and occasionally reverse bone loss—especially when part of a balanced diet and exercise regimen. Since bones are made mostly of calcium, it's tempting to believe that calcium is the most potent thing we can take to prevent bone loss, but it's not—at least, not by itself. In most cases, other therapies—such as estrogen replacement or those using bisphos-phonates or SERMs—are needed to adjust the way the body handles calcium.

CALCIUM AND PARATHYROID HORMONE

The success of estrogen replacement therapy has now been satisfacto-rily explained by the discovery of estrogen receptors on osteoblasts and by the clear demonstration that bone resorption agents are stimulated by estrogen loss. With this knowledge on the one hand and the dra-matic effectiveness of hormone replacement on the other, the scientific community came to accept that the principal cause of osteoporosis was menopausal estrogen loss. Estrogen replacement was for many years the only effective treatment of any sort for anyone. There were no options for men suffering from osteoporosis and no serious study of their risk for bone loss. It became increasingly common to hear osteo-porosis described as a woman's disease, even though a good one-fifth of those suffering from the disease were men. The prevailing attitude went largely without challenge. Indeed, to this day the FDA has not approved a single medication for osteoporosis in older men, although an increasing number of clinical trials are beginning to focus on men. Still, it is not really surprising that the dramatic effectiveness of estro-gen replacement therapy led most scientists and doctors to believe that the major cause of osteoporosis was menopausal estrogen loss.

With the benefit of hindsight, it is now easy to see that these con-clusions were premature. Postmenopausal estrogen deficiency is an important factor in osteoporosis, but not the only one. Osteoporosis caused by corticosteroid excess, poor diet, and immobilization (those who are bed-ridden) still requires explanation. And although meno-pause affects women all over the world in very much the same way, patterns of bone loss and osteoporosis vary significantly from place to place and race to race. Also, premenopausal bone loss is by no means rare, and there is no doubt that men lose bone mass in a way that leads to the same type of fracture complications as women.

Researchers in Japan led by Dr. Takuo Fujita theorize that calcium deficiency and secondary hyperparathyroidism (overactivity of the parathyroid glands) are a normal course of events in elderly women and men. Primary hyperparathyroidism is caused by a disorder of the glands themselves. Secondary hyperparathyroidism is triggered by low levels of calcium in the blood, which are themselves the result of a calcium-deficient diet, poor intestinal absorption, or both. In order to maintain adequate blood calcium for calcium's important metabolic functions, parathyroid hormone (PTH) is released. This stimulates the activity of osteoclasts, which promptly break down bone and release calcium and phosphate into the blood. Scientists use blood PTH levels as a useful indicator of calcium metabolism.

A study in 1979 compared the rates of osteoporosis in two populations in two different areas of Yugoslavia, one with low calcium intake, one with high. The results established a clear connection between calcium and osteoporosis. It seems incredible today that calcium loss was first considered as a cause of osteoporosis only in 1960—the Yugoslavia study was the first to confirm it.

Estrogen helps the intestines absorb calcium. It also aids the final conversion by the kidneys of vitamin D into its active state, which enhances calcium absorption even more. The marker that scientists look for is the relative absence of circulating parathyroid hormone, which normally increases in response to low blood-calcium levels. Other researchers achieved the same fall in PTH secretion using calcium supplementation alone, showing that calcium therapy can be a viable alternative to estrogen therapy. However, doses as high as 2,400 mg per day were required. Not everybody can respond to these doses, especially the elderly.

Dr. Fujita's team began to focus on factors affecting absorption, including both the metabolic activity of calcium in the intestines and the mechanical properties of the calcium preparation. It is known that the effect of calcium depends upon how much is absorbed, up to a certain threshold. For example, those suffering from acute deficiency respond more effectively to calcium supplementation than those suffering from more moderate declines. Somehow, their ability to absorb the calcium is enhanced.

Other factors affect this threshold. Calcium taken with food is more efficiently absorbed than on an empty stomach. And calcium citrate is more easily absorbed than calcium carbonate. Could even greater absorbability provoke a more effective response? The Japanese researchers attempted to shift this threshold by developing different, more absorbable forms of calcium, theorizing that "a good calcium preparation that penetrates the intestinal barrier may change the threshold and exert effects otherwise unexpected in conventional calcium preparations."

The result is a particularly absorbable calcium source—absorbable algal calcium (AAA Ca—see chapter 5). It has shown great promise in suppressing secondary hyperparathyroidism, in which parathyroid hormone stimulates osteoclasts to break down bone.

The secondary hyperparathyroidism of old age upsets this balance and leads to excessive osteoclast activity and overall bone loss, with a flood of calcium into the blood. Bone is not the only part of the body to suffer as a result of this activity. From the bloodstream, the calcium passes through the kidneys (where in sufficient concentrations it may cause kidney stones) and then into the urine and out of the body. The remainder is deposited in soft tissue, such as blood vessels and the brain, where it contributes to functional deterioration of various organs, leading to hypertension, arteriosclerosis, diabetes, and senile dementia. Deposits in and around mobile joints also contribute to osteoarthritis.

Traditionally, osteoporosis and osteoarthritis were seen as mutually exclusive disorders—the first characterized by too little calcium, the second by too much. The theory that they stem from a single event is, at face value, paradoxical, which is why Dr. Fujita has termed this theory the Calcium Paradox. As a therapy for hyperparathyroidism, calcium taken in sufficient quantities prevents osteoporosis, but not simply by building bones. Rather, it preempts parathyroid hormone secretion and prevents the body from depleting our great store of skeletal calcium by restoring hormonal balance.

TYPES OF CALCIUM

The calcium we obtain from foods or supplement pills is not elemental (simple) calcium, but a calcium salt. In this form, calcium is compounded with other elements that make the whole digestible. Calcium carbonate and calcium citrate are two examples. Each chemical compound of calcium has a distinctive proportion of elemental calcium. You must take two or three times as much calcium citrate as calcium carbonate to get the same net dose of elemental calcium. Read the label carefully to see whether the amount mentioned refers to size of the pill or the amount of elemental calcium.

Our ability to digest calcium (or as we more commonly say, the calcium's absorbability) is determined by the availability of vitamin D and also in part by the physical qualities of the calcium preparation. Since only a small fraction of the calcium we eat actually makes it into our blood, this is an important factor and is the focus of the current search for new calcium sources. Calcium carbonate taken as part of a meal is more efficiently absorbed than when taken independently, and chewable calcium carbonate is generally more absorbable than calcium carbonate pills.

Many forms of calcium are combined with vitamin D. It is not a good idea to rely blindly on the manufacturer's dosage. Your body probably can't get too much calcium, but it can certainly get too much vitamin D. If you are taking lots of calcium, check the packaging and make sure you're taking no more than 600 IU per day of vitamin D. You'll save money, too.

In a clinical trial of elderly women, supplementation of calcium was reported to inhibit zinc absorption, so it may be prudent to supplement this element as well. According to estimates from this study, you will need about 8 mg of zinc for each 600 mg of calcium.

Some sources of calcium, notably dolomite and bone meal, may contain lead. These products should be avoided by children and breastfeeding mothers. Some oyster shell products may also contain heavy metals (see p. 92 for more information). If you cannot be sure of the purity of a particular calcium product, it's best to avoid it, especially considering the large doses that are required to maintain health.

Recommended intake of calcium in infants and preadolescent children runs from 200 to 1,000 mg per day. Adolescents and young adults require about 1,200 to 1,400 mg per day. Adults and seniors will net 1,500 and up. A total daily amount of 2,400 is not unusual.

Calcium Carbonate

Calcium carbonate is the oldest and most available source of supplemental calcium. The differences among various formulations have to do with solubility, and the variability from one product to another is quite alarming; some are virtually insoluble. Look for the USP (U.S. Pharmacopeia) logo on the bottle for a respectable product. If you're still not sure, drop a pill in a glass of warm water. If it doesn't start to dissolve within ten minutes, it's not much use to you or your bones.

Chewable calcium formulations are best, such as those sold as antacids (over-the-counter indigestion medications). If you often suffer from indigestion, it may make you feel a little better to know that high stomach acidity aids calcium absorption. On the other hand, if you do not suffer from excess stomach acid and take calcium on an empty stomach, your stomach may react by becoming acidic. Your daily intake should be split into at least two doses, morning and evening, and preferably taken with meals. Don't forget that lots of roughage (fibrous foods) will carry much of the calcium straight into the stool. Doctors today routinely prescribe regimens of one to three grams (1,000–3,000 mg) of calcium per day, which is quite a lot for the intestines to handle. The older we get, the more difficult it becomes.

Supplemented calcium carbonate can cause constipation. If you experience this, take smaller, more frequent doses, always with meals or at least some food. Twenty percent of people in their seventies suffer from atrophic gastritis (age-related inflammation of the stomach lining) and are completely unable to absorb calcium carbonate except with meals. This figure doubles among eighty-year-olds and climbs with age. An alternative is calcium citrate, a more absorbable salt of calcium.

Calcium carbonate contains about 40 percent elemental calcium.

Calcium Citrate (Calcium Citrate-Malate)

Calcium citrate is much more absorbable than calcium carbonate but contains only about half as much elemental calcium, so it is taken in larger quantities. In spite of the great importance given to absorbability and the undisputed fact that calcium citrate is so much more absorbable, the only large, randomized trial comparing these two preparations revealed no significant differences in bone health between people taking calcium carbonate and those using calcium citrate. It is generally better tolerated but is also more expensive. Manufacturers recommend taking it on an empty stomach with water or a citrus juice.

Calcium citrate contains about 20 percent elemental calcium.

Other Calcium Salts

Calcium gluconate contains barely 9 percent elemental calcium. To get 500 mg of elemental calcium, you would have to swallow five and a half grams of calcium gluconate—several handfuls of pills. Calcium lactate contains 13 percent elemental calcium. Calcium phosphate dibasic is about 23 percent calcium and tricalcium phosphate is about 39 percent elemental calcium.

Vitamin D

Calcium needs help to cross through cell membranes, especially from the gastrointestinal tract into the bloodstream. For this reason, consuming it is only half the battle. Getting it from your intestines into the bloodstream becomes an increasingly uphill task as we grow older. Even at the best of times we absorb barely 30 percent of our dietary supply of calcium, and excrete the remainder.

Vitamin D is the key to calcium absorption. That is why it is frequently added to calcium supplements and also to milk—our oldest and most traditional source of calcium. Vitamin D deficiency in children leads to rickets, and in adults to osteomalacia—both bone-softening diseases that affect the way calcium and other minerals coalesce into bone. These diseases are easily treated by vitamin D supplementation.

Still, vitamin D supplementation is not necessarily enough to solve the problem of bone loss leading to osteoporosis.

In North America, vitamin D deficiency is uncommon but not unknown. Fifteen minutes or so of direct sunlight on your face, arms, and shoulders per day enables your skin to produce adequate supplies of vitamin D. However, sunscreens or even a thin pane of glass can block this effect of sunlight. People in northern climates, especially immobile people or those living in nursing homes, may suffer from inadequate exposure to sunlight. Studies carried out in London, England, showed that Middle Eastern women who traditionally cover their entire bodies and heads often exhibit vitamin D deficiency when living in this northern city, particularly during the winter with its very short, often overcast days.

That vitamin D is important to bone metabolism is beyond doubt; however, its precise mechanism is complex and has not yet been fully explained. We know it serves at least two important functions—intestinal absorption of calcium and stimulation of osteoclast (and perhaps also osteoblast) activity. We know it follows a lively path through the body. It begins its journey in the stomach from dietary sources, or in the skin where it is synthesized by sunlight from a particular form of cholesterol (7-dehydrocholesterol). In either case, at this point it is called pre–vitamin D. As it is passes through the liver it is transformed into 25 hydroxy-vitamin D_3, the most abundant form of vitamin D in the body, but still not the end product. Only after the kidneys have broken it down to its active form— calcitriol (1,25 dihydroxy-vitamin D)—does it aid calcium absorption.

A supplement pill is normally enough to restore adequate vitamin D levels in those who are deficient, but the body's own regulating mechanism—parathyroid hormone—will kick in too. The secretion of this hormone drives the kidneys to manufacture more calcitriol. Of course, this depends on the presence of the dietary or skin-manufactured pre–vitamin D. In either case, the release of parathyroid hormone also stimulates osteoclasts (bone-dissolving cells) at a time when calcium absorption is already impaired. Because the intestines cannot under these circumstances provide adequate calcium to the blood, more parathyroid hormone is released, drawing calcium from bone for essential heart and nerve functions. There is no knowing how much calcium may be lost before this vicious cycle resolves itself, if indeed it does.

Direct supplementation with calcitriol, which requires no further transformation in order to act directly on bone, is a potent way to increase calcium absorption. However, this has been known to raise calcium blood levels too much, resulting in hypercalcemia (abnormally high calcium levels), characterized by nausea, vomiting, lethargy, depression, thirst, kidney stones, and excessive urination. Calcitriol is not a benign drug, and long-term use may damage the kidneys. Advanced cases may result in extreme fatigue and muscle weakness. If you exhibit symptoms of hypercalcemia, your doctor may order tests of both kidney and liver levels of vitamin D.

Calcium supplementation is only effective when accompanied by healthy vitamin D levels, and vitamin D supplementation is only effective on people deficient in vitamin D. Those with liver or kidney disease may be unable to metabolize vitamin D effectively. Also, some antiseizure medication will increase the speed at which the body eliminates it. And aging is characterized by falling vitamin D levels in the kidneys.

Vitamin D studies have also led to genetic explanations for the onset of osteoporosis. Certain cells have vitamin D receptors, providing a biochemical anchor that enables it to get to work. Some people are born with a genetic imperfection in this receptor (called BB) and are at particular risk for osteoporosis. Still, there is reason to believe that regular supplementation of calcium and vitamin D may be enough to override this particular vulnerability.

Vitamin K_2

Vitamin K_2 is needed in the extracellular matrix of bone where it plays a part in the formation of osteocalcin, a bone protein. The role of osteocalcin is not clear, but it may play a part in bone resorption. Vitamin K_2

is found readily in green leafy vegetables. If you eat a cupful of lettuce or other greens each day, vitamin K_2 supplementation is unnecessary. In excessive amounts, laboratory-synthesized vitamin K_2 can cause jaundice (yellowing of the skin).

Treating Fractures

In recent years, for the first time, restorative therapies have become available to patients with osteoporotic fractures. A procedure known as vertebroplasty has been developed at the Mayo Clinic. It is a mechanical treatment involving the injection of bone cement into vertebrae damaged by compression fracture. It results in more stable bone and diminished pain. It gets people on their feet and gives them back some independence at a time when they might otherwise be tempted to give up hope, become increasingly depressed, and fade away.

In percutaneous vertebroplasty, a needle is inserted into the body of the vertebra and the cement—a polymethyl-methylacrylate—is injected into the bone. The existing fracture and deformation is not repaired, but the bone is nevertheless reinforced, strengthening the spine as a whole. Up to four vertebrae at a time have been treated in this way with reports of mild to significant relief of pain and improved mobility. This procedure is usually carried out in the lower spine, where fractures are more common and vertebrae are larger and more accessible. It is more difficult in the upper vertebrae but also less necessary since fractures tend to appear first in the lower spine, which bears greater weight.

A Case Study of Advanced Osteoporosis

Jackie is seventy-three and still works part-time. Her menopause began at age fifty and she was started on hormone replacement therapy, but she was afraid of developing breast cancer and quit after barely three years.

In the last decade and a half Jackie has fractured many bones, including her left hip, right wrist, and right elbow. She has also recently suffered numerous vertebral compression fractures and has lost two to three inches in height. Jackie is a small, thin woman, under five feet tall and weighing under 100 pounds. Her thyroid examination revealed no abnormalities. Her back showed severe curvature both backward and sideways (kyphosis and scoliosis).

She and her gynecologist sat down to determine the factors that had contributed to her condition. As a teenager she had smoked for a brief period before quitting. She never drank alcohol, nor has she ever used glucocorticoids, anticonvulsants, or thyroid medications. Her mother fractured her hip twice, with complications that ultimately led to her death, but there was no family history of breast cancer. Her daily diet contained about 300 mg of calcium. She had never had kidney stones. Jackie also has problems with high blood pressure and heart disease. She had had bypass surgery twice, and a cancerous kidney had been successfully removed.

The doctor sent her for blood tests and a bone-density study. Scans were made of her hip, including the neck and head of the thigh bone. Laboratory results suggested normal levels of both osteoclast and osteoblast activity, providing no hint of her condition. However, collagen breakdown values were elevated, suggesting increased bone resorption. Her BMD results were very low, and several spinal compression fractures were evident on X-rays.

Compared with women with a similar low bone mass and no fractures, Jackie's history places her at even greater risk for future fractures. Because she discontinued HRT so soon after menopause, it is unlikely that she derived much benefit from it. Moreover, she is white, thin, and has a brief history of smoking in her teenage years. Because of her history of coronary artery disease, she avoids cheese, a rich source of dietary calcium, and dislikes milk. Although she has no history of elevated blood calcium levels, kidney tumors are known to stimulate the activity of parathyroid hormone, which promotes bone loss.

Jackie was diagnosed with severe postmenopausal osteoporosis. In addition to her heart medication and a cholesterol-lowering drug, she now takes folic acid, vitamins B_6 and B_{12}, aspirin, vitamin E, a multi-vitamin supplement, and 1,200 mg of calcium carbonate per day. The doctor added vitamin D and D_3 supplements and suggested she take up walking as a daily exercise, which she has done. She was also given alendronate to inhibit further bone resorption. Finally, the doctor ordered a repeat bone densitometry one or two years later to determine the effectiveness of these steps.

Jackie's daughters also are at risk for osteoporosis because of their strong family history of fractures. Their BMD and fracture risk should be assessed at menopause so that preventive treatment can be begun when its potential benefits are greatest.

Conclusion

Estrogen replacement therapy was the first effective treatment for one of the most dramatic forms of bone loss, and certainly the most widespread—postmenopausal estrogen deficiency. However, some women on estrogen became particularly prone to cancer of the uterine lining, and there are fears that estrogen may also promote breast cancer. Selective estrogen receptor modulators offer estrogenlike effects without its risks, and calcitonin is particularly suited to the elderly and even those with existing osteoporosis. Meanwhile, it has become clear that estrogen deficiency is but one cause of osteoporosis and that other treatments are necessary for both women and men. Bisphosphonates offer a different approach to the maintenance of bone, and alendronate seems protective of male bones. Curiously, the role of calcium is still not fully understood. Its importance in the prevention and treatment of osteoporosis may lie more in its ability to maintain blood-calcium levels and prevent parathyroid-induced bone resorption than in its use in building bone.

5

Alternative
Therapies

This chapter discusses therapies not in current use by conventional health practitioners. Some are exciting, but they haven't yet entered mainstream use. Some are considered erroneous by scientists but are nevertheless still available.

The most interesting therapy described in this chapter uses active absorbable algal calcium (AAA Ca), a new calcium source developed in Japan as an adjunct to the Calcium Paradox theory of bone loss. Phytoestrogens are an important option for women afraid of or in danger of osteoporosis. They are used as a natural hormone therapy. We also discuss human growth hormone and melatonin, natural sources of vitamin D, and other mineral and vitamin sources used in the prevention and treatment of osteoporosis.

Like any other medical intervention, alternative therapies can have undesirable effects. If you choose to follow one or more of these treatments, you must consult an experienced practitioner. This person should help you determine the appropriate remedy, dose, and schedule and tell you what to watch out for. If on top of that you wish to continue conventional treatment, you must at all costs tell your doctor about the other therapies you are following.

Don't make the mistake of thinking that so-called "natural" therapies are inherently harmless. Nothing could be further from the truth. Any substance potent enough to affect bone renewal will affect your metabolism, and such interventions always pose a risk of certain imbalances. Natural products are as likely to interact with one another and with pharmaceutical drugs as any other molecule, sometimes with unexpected results.

Active Absorbable Algal Calcium (AAA Ca)

Active absorbable algae calcium (AAA Ca, or triple-A calcium) is a combination of heated oyster shell and a heated algal ingredient (HAI). It is available in North America under the trade name AdvaCal. The oyster shell is powdered and then heated in a vacuum to approximately 900° C, so that its constituent calcium carbonate is rendered into calcium oxide and calcium hydroxide, both highly absorbable. To this is added an acid extract of the seaweed cystophyllum fusiforme, heated under reduced pressure at 800° C. A number of clinical human trials have repeatedly demonstrated the exceptional absorbability of this product. Its high proportion of elemental calcium is another advantage.

Calcium carbonate is the most common of all calcium salts, but the calcium carbonate in oyster shell is different from other sources. Although it has the same chemical composition ($CaCO_3$), its mechanical properties differ. It is arranged in a unique spatial arrangement—a lamellar crystalline structure (built of fine overlapping scales)—which, researchers theorize, may contribute to the solubility and bioavailability (usefulness to the body) of the final product.

Even though AAA Ca is subjected to high temperatures, the residual product also contains trace amounts of the amino acids serine, glycine, proline, and leucine, measured in thousandths of a milligram per gram of the rendered oyster shell. The heated algal ingredient adds three more amino acids in similar concentrations: histidine, tyrosine, and valine. It is known that certain amino acids will help the body absorb calcium more efficiently, but the amounts found here are microscopic, and scientists would not normally expect to witness any significant bioactivity. Nevertheless, the heated oyster shell's great absorbability has been repeatedly demonstrated, and researchers claim that the addition of the heated algal ingredient enhances its absorbability even more.

This product was recently developed in Japan, where it has been subjected to a large number of clinical trials. These were carried out under the supervision of Dr. Takuo Fujita, president of the Japan Osteoporosis Foundation and director of the Calcium Research Institute. After having published over four hundred scientific papers on calcium in peer-review journals, this lifelong researcher formulated the Calcium Paradox theory of osteoporosis (see chapter 1). Once the high absorbability of AAA Ca had been established, he used it to test his theory.

AAA Calcium was initially tested for biovailability—which in this case means the degree to which it is absorbed through the intestine and the effect it has on parathyroid hormone levels. In initial tests, subjects were given a 1,000-mg dose of either calcium carbonate or AAA Calcium, and their urine was tested two hours later. Results suggested that AAA Ca was more absorbable. Following that, a two-year randomized, prospective, double-blind trial was carried out on a group of elderly women (average age, eighty years). All were given 900-mg-per-day doses of AAA Ca, calcium carbonate, or placebo (sugar pill). Changes in lumbar spine BMD were measured in all groups and the first was found to benefit the most, actually increasing bone-mineral density very significantly. Measurements of parathyroid hormone (PTH) and alkaline phosphatase were taken regularly. Low PTH levels confirmed that elevated calcium levels were suppressing PTH secretion, and elevated levels of alkaline phosphatase confirmed an increase in bone formation.

The researchers concluded that secondary hyperparathyroidism is an inevitable consequence of aging—as long as we live long enough— and that it can be suppressed by maintaining calcium levels with the highly absorbable AAA Ca. Their suggestion is that by maintaining good blood-calcium balance, the flooding of calcium into soft tissue is also avoided and the risk of other Calcium Paradox diseases (see chapter 1) is diminished.

Having established the effectiveness of AAA Ca, researchers went on to determine the best dosing schedule. In a group of nine healthy male volunteers, it was found that those taking 150 mg after each meal plus 450 mg at bedtime experienced lower nighttime PTH levels (when they reach their peak) than others taking 300 mg after each meal alone.

Additionally, Triple-A calcium does not contain heavy metals. It seems to modify the intestinal and metabolic response to calcium and parathyroid hormone, restoring a positive balance to bone renewal without the use of hormones or pharmaceutical drugs.

Phytoestrogens

Phytoestrogens are natural estrogenlike compounds known as isoflavones and lignans. They are derived from several plant sources, including most commonly the seeds of soybeans and flaxseed. Their concentration in these foods varies enormously depending on the seed's genetic makeup, where it was grown, and the environmental conditions during growth.

Phytoestrogens are not identical to the human hormone but may act in similar, though weaker, ways to counter bone loss and heart disease. Most doctors feel that their effects have not been adequately studied in clinical trials, but they are generally accepted to have weak antiestrogenic effects in breast tissue—which is one of the main attractions, even though the link between breast cancer and estrogen is controversial. Phytoestrogens are obtainable in many countries without prescription and also appeal to those who prefer vegetable-based therapies to animal or pharmaceutical sources.

Most doctors are reluctant to prescribe a regimen of phytoestrogens. First of all, their action is very weak and unpredictable. There is no reason to believe that these natural remedies are inherently better or less troublesome than conventional ones. Like estrogen, phytoestrogens have been linked to endometrial hyperplasia (overgrowth of cells of the uterine lining).

Both pharmaceutical sources of estrogen and phytoestrogen products are formulated in the laboratory, and there is no scientific evidence to support the notion that plant sources offer more benefits or fewer risks than animal sources. In fact, the one thing we know for sure about phytoestrogens is that they must be taken in large doses in order to promote any significant estrogenic effects.

Many scientists will say that eating foods said to be high in phytoestrogens is unlikely to affect your levels of circulating hormones, because they are derived in the laboratory by complex processes that your body cannot duplicate. However, studies at the University of Illinois suggest that large quantities of dietary soy protein may play a role in maintaining bone health. Although there is not enough evidence as yet to convince the medical establishment of the bone-protecting powers of soy, there is certainly not enough evidence to discount it, either.

Vitamin D

Vitamin D is found abundantly in cod-liver oil and is also available in other seafoods such as raw herring, salmon, and sardines in oil. Eggs, chicken liver, Swiss cheese, milk, and margarine also provide vitamin D. Whether you take your vitamin D as food supplements or by careful dietary planning, it is important that you take the right amount. Too much vitamin D can cause hypercalcemia (abnormally high calcium levels in the blood) and lead to nausea, vomiting, lethargy, depression, thirst, and excessive urination. Advanced cases may result in extreme fatigue and muscle weakness. However, reports of various dosing schedules for vitamin D vary widely in their effects. Consult your doctor to determine a dose appropriate for your condition.

Soy Beans

Studies carried out by the Division of Nutritional Science at the University of Illinois found that women who ate large amounts of soy had stronger bones.

Progesterone Cream for Men

Progesterone cream is an established therapy for women and is usually used for dryness and other disorders of the vagina. Its use in men is not a common practice, but it has been popularly promoted as a restorative of weakened libido. Progesterone cream has negligible effects on bone-mineral density in women and there is no reason to believe that it will be any more useful for men's bones.

Human Growth Hormone

Human growth hormone (HGH) is secreted throughout or lives, not just while we're growing up. However, like most other secretions of the endocrine (hormonal) system, HGH levels dwindle as we get older. Clinical trials and experiments with HGH to date have mostly been concerned with childhood disorders caused by HGH deficiency, and possible treatments with its clinical replacement. A few trials have documented the effects of HGH supplementation in healthy or osteoporotic adults. Some doctors are experimenting with HGH as an antiaging therapy, and the FDA in 1996 approved its use for long-term replacement therapy in adults with growth hormone deficiency.

HGH was originally obtained from the brains of human cadavers, and was extremely expensive. Today, less expensive laboratory formulations are available, as are secretagogues—simple, inexpensive amino acids that can increase growth hormone secretion. Stories about HGH sometimes describe spectacular results, including regrowth of age-shrunken organs, the return to elderly people of 20:20 vision, the regrowth of lost hair, and even the return of faded pigment. But no long-term scientific studies have been carried out, and reliable information is hard to come by. Most doctors are skeptical of claims made about HGH and, even if they find the stories believable, are uneasy about using it. Long-term consequences are completely unknown and difficult to predict. Side effects are said to include fluid retention, joint pain, diabetes, and high blood pressure. Unsubstantiated reports that consistently elevated HGH levels encourage the growth of cancer also circulate freely. In fact, the debate has become emotionally charged. HGH works at a fundamental level of the endocrine (hormonal) system and seems to affect most glands and organs in the body, sometimes with dramatic results. These claims are extraordinary. But, say skeptics, so might be the long-term, negative consequences.

The idea that HGH encourages bone growth is quite believable. After all, it affects many metabolic functions, starting with most of the glands of the endocrine system. HGH is said to restore glands and internal organs to their youthful size and functionality. It builds muscle in elderly people without exercise, and with exercise promotes a response normally only witnessed in the young.

Swedish researchers have found evidence that HGH stimulates osteoblast (bone regrowth) activity. They have also described the regrowth and strengthening of vertebrae in elderly people with a measurable improvement in BMD, protein synthesis in the bone, and growth of the intervertebral disks in the spine, leading to restored height.

Even though HGH replacement therapy remains strictly controlled in the United States and Canada, HGH modulation is now freely available to anyone purchasing over-the-counter HGH secretagogues (promoters of HGH secretion) such as the amino acids arginine and glutamine.

Melatonin

Recent studies in Japan have tested the use of melatonin on bone formation. Melatonin is secreted by the pineal gland and is known to control daily body rhythms—it is used by some people to counteract jet lag. Large doses (1 percent of total diet) also appear to build strong bones in laboratory rats without affecting the growth rate, size of internal organs, or serum levels of calcium and phosphorus. Much research remains to be carried out on melatonin. It significantly influences the entire endocrine (hormonal) system, and its long-term effects, especially when taken in large doses, are quite unknown.

DHEA—Testosterone Precursor

Declining hormone levels in aging men have led to the use of testosterone therapy to relieve problems of waning strength and reduced sex drive. DHEA (dehydroepiandrosterone) is a precursor (building block) of testosterone that is sometimes promoted as a way to elevate testosterone levels. Unfortunately, before it can take part in testosterone synthesis it is altered by the digestive system and does not produce the desired response. In fact, high doses of DHEA seem to depress testosterone levels. If you think you need testosterone replacement, consult your doctor.

Wild Yams (Sweet Potato)

Wild yams produce a compound that is used by the pharmaceutical industry to produce progesterones, so some people advocate eating yams as part of a natural hormone replacement therapy. Unfortunately, the human body does not operate like a pharmaceutical laboratory—at least, not in this case. Yams are a perfectly good food, but eating them is not like taking progesterone, just as eating soybean seed, flaxseed, and other natural sources of phytoestrogens does not constitute estrogen replacement therapy.

Experimental Developments

Experimental research in biotechnology is revolutionizing the study of osteoporosis just as it is transforming the world of medicine in general. This section briefly presents some late-breaking developments. Some may lead to dead ends. Others may promote advances years or—more probably—decades in the future.

A new compound developed recently at Washington University in St. Louis, Missouri—called by the experimental name SC56631— blocks the receptor in bone that is normally used by osteoclasts to attach to and break down bone. By preventing old bone from being broken down as usual, the compound slows or stops bone loss. However, if osteoclasts cannot do their job, neither perhaps can osteoblasts, which normally move into the footsteps of osteoclasts to build new bone. Questions remain to be answered. Still, this might lead to a short-term therapy to rebuild bone quickly and prevent fractures.

A rare genetic mutation that results in weak teeth and strong bone may also hold clues for scientists seeking new therapies. The disease caused by this mutation is called tricho-dento-osseous. It results in little or no tooth enamel and often painful, unsightly and diseased teeth. However, it also builds extraordinarily strong bones that rarely fracture or break—even in severe automobile accidents. Researchers at the University of North Carolina are studying this defect hoping it may lead to new understanding of bone mineral density.

Another advance is the identification of a gene essential to the formation of bone. The discovery that normal skeletal development depends on two active copies of the gene Cbfa1 is expected to open doors to new avenues of research.

It has been recently recognized that estrogen can induce programmed cell death in osteoclasts. This understanding has provoked a hunt for other compounds with similar estrogenlike functions. This may lead to drug therapies that can more effectively slow osteoclast activity (bone breakdown) and restore bone renewal to a state of balance.

A study at Colorado State University has developed a novel approach to bone health. Sheep regularly subjected to subtle but high-frequency vibration in their hind legs were found to increase their bone density by an average of 3 percent. Half of the sheep were constrained so that they stood on a vibrating metal plate for twenty minutes a day, five days a week for a year. The researches believe the vibration stimulates bone growth in ways similar to exercise. This may become a useful therapy for bedridden people and others unable to exercise adequately.

PARATHYROID HORMONE

We have seen that parathyroid hormone is often responsible for the removal of excessive calcium from bones. This occurs particularly among sufferers of primary hyperparathyroidism (a disorder of the parathyroid gland itself) or in elderly people who frequently—some say inevitably—suffer from secondary hyperparathyroidism (excessive levels of parathyroid hormone triggered by low blood-calcium levels). Although parathyroid hormone stimulates the bone-resorption activity of osteoclasts and initiates bone breakdown, the sites it creates attract osteoblasts (bone renewal agents), which renew the bone. Clinical trials have been performed with parathyroid hormone therapy to adjust the balance of bone breakdown and renewal with a view to improving overall bone-mineral density.

Studies carried out at the Yale School of Medicine found that when used alone, intermittent daily injections of PTH under the skin resulted in consistent gains in trabecular (inner) bone, although the effects on the cortical (outer) shell of bones was less effective. This approach is now being tested in combination with estrogen therapy. Whether this will lead to a PTH-based therapy or simply reveal the role of PTH in bone loss more clearly is uncertain. Similar research into the role of PTH is being carried out at various institutions.

Researchers in Switzerland working on animal models discovered that parathyroid hormone receptors are found on osteoblasts but not osteoclasts. Nevertheless, PTH indirectly affects osteoclasts, increasing their number and activity. They found that intermittent rather than continuous administration of PTH was needed to produce its anabolic (protein-building) activity in bone.

In other animal trials conducted in New York, researchers tested the combination of PTH therapy with estrogen and separately with alendronate (a bisphosphonate, see chapter 4) and concluded that such combination therapies for postmenopausal women with osteoporosis warranted further investigation.

Further studies at the University of California in San Diego show great promise for this therapy, but recent studies in rats linked high doses of parathyroid hormone to a risk for a malignant bone tumor called osteogenic carcinoma. Although this disorder is rare in humans and has not been observed in human subjects undergoing PTH therapy, it is seen as a signal to proceed cautiously.

Many of the therapies designed to slow bone loss and prevent osteoporosis focus on inhibiting the function of osteoclasts. However, these bone-dissolving cells perform a vital function, preparing the ground for incoming osteoblasts and renewed bone. A true long-term bone therapy must address the entire bone renewal cycle, and PTH is a promising area for research.

Conclusion

The therapies described in this chapter have been suggested as alternatives to traditional therapies, which often rely on pharmaceutical drugs and hormonal preparations. While conventional remedies have been greatly successful and have prevented osteoporosis in countless women, the search for less invasive and more general therapies continues. The emergence of a theory of osteoporosis that addresses men as well as women and the development of new calcium preparations is good news. Also, ongoing research into parathyroid hormone therapies promises new drugs and new approaches to osteoporosis.

6

The Osteoporosis
Remedy: Prevention

It's never too early to begin thinking about osteoporosis prevention. Despite the fact that people think it is a disease of old age, the ideal time to begin a prevention program is before bone loss starts to occur, in your late twenties, or thirties at the latest.

If you are young and healthy, you must prevent bone loss as much as possible. If you are osteopenic, you must try to rebuild bone. If you are osteoporotic, you must avoid falls that may easily cause fractures. In other words, to prevent osteoporosis from dominating your life, you must understand your current bone condition and most significant risk factors. Most of us are subject to impaired calcium absorption and secondary hyperparathyroidism as we age, and almost all women are at risk of postmenopausal bone loss. But there are many other possible factors, some of them constituting lifelong risks.

Assuming that certain drugs or supplements will help you as effectively as the next person is bad planning. Genetic, environmental, and lifestyle factors may be enough to tip the balance. If you embark on a preventive therapy that only poorly or indirectly addresses your needs, you may continue to lose bone while under the pleasant delusion that you are safe from osteoporosis. Just as osteoporosis is a silent killer, the effectiveness of preventive measures is also silent. You can only tell how well you're doing by going for periodic BMD tests.

There are dozens of possible ways to prevent the loss of bone mineral density and the onset of osteoporosis. Taking calcium and vitamin D is generally preventive and may be all you need—although there are dozens of reasons why you might be unable to absorb enough of these minerals. There's no guarantee that any particular method will slow bone loss sufficiently, or that your choice of calcium supplement or the way you take it is appropriate for your digestive system.

Going to your doctor is an important step in preventive therapy. Ask for a BMD test and discuss all possible options based on your own medical records. If you are a woman, estrogen therapy or SERMs might well be your final choice. For both men and women, bisphosphonates and highly absorbable calcium supplements like triple-A calcium offer promising alternatives.

Nevertheless, without question, the best preventive measure is exercise. Under ideal circumstances, exercise preempts the need for hormonal supplements by raising your body's metabolism to its most efficient levels. It primes the cardiovascular system, stimulates the endocrine system, and reminds your body that you are alive. It's a 100 percent natural treatment.

Exercise

The best thing you can do for your bones is also the best thing you can do for your body, mind, and morale—exercise. The worst thing you can do is the Western world's most widespread and reckless indulgence—nothing at all. The truth is, our modern lifestyle has made us soft. To stay in shape, we must go out of our way to develop and follow a fitness schedule. Today exercise is optional—no longer an inescapable part of life, as it was for our ancestors, whose survival depended on physical strength.

Many modern conveniences contribute to our sedentary lifestyle. The epitome of labor-saving devices is the automobile, which saves us the labor of walking and deprives us of the one weight-bearing exercise we can all use. Young or old, strong boned or osteoporotic, walking is the best way to keep up bone mineral density in your legs and hips. Even those with existing fractures should walk as much as they can. Surrendering to osteoporosis and losing mobility drain the bones even more quickly. Nevertheless, if you are osteopenic or osteoporotic, you must consult a licensed physiotherapist rather than a fitness trainer. If your skeleton is either weak or damaged, some types of movement may worsen your condition, and the physiotherapist will suggest therapeutic exercises unknown to a fitness trainer.

A little exercise is better than none and frequent, regular exercise is even better, although there is such a thing as excess. You can benefit in many ways by going beyond the minimum and you might even enjoy it. Regular exercise brings a tangible sense of well-being and a natural endorphin high. It improves breathing and blood circulation, increases energy levels and makes most people feel better about themselves. And if you do it well, it builds better bones at any age.

We know this by comparing BMD studies of two groups at opposite ends of the exercise spectrum—highly inactive and highly active young people. The results tell a vivid story.

In studies in the 1970s and 1980s, healthy young men who were suddenly and completely bedridden for long periods were seen to lose bone-mineral density at an alarming rate. Losses in BMD of 0.5 percent per month to 0.9 percent per week were recorded consistently. It was no surprise that they lost bone—the theory that bones respond to exercise or inactivity was formulated over a century ago—but the rate of loss was shocking. It has recently been found, however, that such figures are only seen in cases of absolute bedrest. Those able to manage even the minimal exertion of going to the bathroom under their own power suffered considerably less damage.

Studies at the other end of the scale tell us about the bones of world-class athletes. The vertebral bones of weight lifters are very strong, often in direct proportion to the weights they lift. Soccer players and runners have strong hip and leg bones. So do tennis players, who also have much greater BMD in their racket arms. This leaves no doubt that the benefits of exercise are very specific. Exercise does not promote any significant global metabolic benefits in your bones—if you want to strengthen your back, you must exercise your back, and so on. But you must also work out in a balanced way, paying attention to your whole body.

Swimming, unfortunately, doesn't promote particularly strong bones. Swimmers are supported by water, just as the bones of astronauts are supported weightlessly. In fact, space flight is a very significant risk factor for osteoporosis. Nowadays, astronauts on long space flights regularly practice specific bone-strengthening exercises. Back on Earth, we refer to a such a regimen as impact-loading and/or weight-bearing exercise.

Impact-loading and weight-bearing exercises are without a doubt the best way to rejuvenate bone metabolism and rebuild strong bones. But before you lift any weights you must consult an expert and begin gradually.

Any activity done on your feet will help maintain the muscles and bones of your lower body. Jogging and the darting movements of competitive field-sports impact bones more frequently and intensely than walking or cycling. This is called impact loading, which is good for bones, but can be hard on joints, especially the knees. Weight machines for the lower body help you maintain a challenging stress on your legs and lower back with very little impact.

Remember to incorporate a cardiovascular warmup prior to your weight routine.

CARDIOVASCULAR EXERCISE

A complete exercise regimen works out both your inner organs and your outer body mass. Since the bodily energy you use during exercise depends upon a ready supply of oxygen, you should begin inside, by priming the cardiovascular system.

The cardiovascular system consists of the lungs, heart, and blood vessels. The object of cardiovascular exercise is to raise the heart rate to a certain level and hold it there in a steady, rhythmic way, to exercise the lungs and heart. It also improves oxygenation of the blood and its distribution into the slackest and most distant arteries. It primes each cell in your body with oxygen and prepares it to respond actively to the stress (not distress) of strenuous exercise.

The focus of a cardiovascular warmup is to work out your heart and lungs, so we begin with the large muscles of the legs and back. Nevertheless, no exercise is purely cardiovascular. Walking or running puts impact-loading forces on the bones of your lower body and helps strengthen muscles and bones there.

Gymnasiums have cardiovascular machines for running, cycling, walking, stepping, climbing, and rowing. Pick one and build up a steady pace. Your breathing will deepen and you will experience increased flow of oxygen from the lungs into the blood. The heart rate rises, pumping oxygenated blood through the complex network of arteries and veins. The heart is a sophisticated pump composed mostly of muscle and responds eagerly to regular workouts.

A cardiovascular warmup also prepares the body to deal with waste products. Each cell manufactures its own energy needs by combining oxygen with dietary nutrients. The process of turning these molecules into energy leaves behind waste products—oxyradicals (or free radicals—freely charged, destructive subatomic ions) that cause untold cumulative damage. Free radical damage is increasingly held responsible for many of the ailments of aging—at least for their early onset and rapid progression. By elevating your metabolism, cardiovascular exercise helps your body neutralize free radicals too, provided it has a ready supply of antioxidant nutrients (scavenging molecules that consume free radicals). Most vitamins serve various antioxidant functions in the body. So do many raw and cooked foods.

Target Heart Rate

The goal of a cardiovascular warmup is to raise your heart rate to a specific target level and maintain it there for a good ten to thirty minutes. Some people spend hours on cardiovascular machines to burn fat. This is generally done at a lower heart rate and doesn't have the same effect as a warmup, even though the machine and the bodily movements are the same.

Your target heart rate is a function of age. First, determine your predicted maximum heart rate by subtracting your age from 220. The target heart rate should lie between 70 percent and 90 percent of your maximum. For example, when you are forty, your maximum heart rate is 180 (220–40), and during warmup your heart rate should be within the range of 126 to 162 beats per minute. Regular, sustained exertion like this dramatically improves the efficiency of heart and lungs, replenishes your inner organs, and primes your muscles.

At least two minutes before you are done, you should start to slow down gradually. A sudden drop from your elevated heart rate can distress the body, which is now ready for action. You are warmed up and ready to work your bones.

WEIGHT-BEARING EXERCISE

To tell your bones to grow stronger, you must push them with impact-loading or weight-bearing activity. Once again, it doesn't matter how old you are. If you can lift it, it will make you stronger—as long as you do it right. Weight lifting is a highly artificial activity and you can hurt yourself by trying to lift too much, or even by lifting very little the wrong way. Your body does not instinctively understand good form and must learn it, preferably from an experienced trainer. This is really not something you should attempt to pick up from a book. You need someone to point out the various muscle groups and make sure you identify them as you exercise. Above all, you must learn to distinguish stress from distress so that your workout is good for you.

The skeleton and muscles together form a machine of rigid levers and pliable motors that move at will. They respond to exercise by adapting to the demands placed on them. The bones are a living part of the body and will react like any other part, though more slowly. Bones become stronger as we use weights to stress and flex both muscles and the bones to which they are attached. Free weights and weight machines are not always necessary. Pull-ups, sit-ups, and push-ups use the weight of your body, and also provide benefit. The point is, you're working against gravity. However you do it, regularly stressing (but not distressing) each muscle and bone sends a message telling it to shape up and grow stronger.

Everybody responds to weight-bearing activity, no matter what their age or physical condition. In other words, whatever you can do will help. Don't believe it's too late or not worth the effort. The only alternative is inevitable, continued bone loss. With sufficient determination, even relatively immobile elderly people can get back on their feet. The key, of course, is motivation. To be of long-term use, exercise must be a lifelong activity. It's never too late to start, but once you do, it should be forever. So it's important that you enjoy it. If it always takes a massive act of self-discipline to get to your workout, you probably haven't found the right one for you, and sooner or later you'll want to change or perhaps quit. But that's not an excuse to give up just because you find it hard at the beginning. Once you experience the tangible benefits of regular exercise, your motivation will grow of itself. You may find it addictive.

Bulk

Weight training does not have to make you big. Even slender, toned muscles can be surprisingly strong. Weight training will firm up your muscles and shape your body in any way you want. Whether you build big muscles depends on several factors, the first one being your testosterone (male hormone) levels. Men have much more testosterone and beef up much more quickly and to a much greater extent than women. Certainly some women have more testosterone than others, but it takes a great deal of effort to build bulging muscles. Nobody has to.

Any sort of muscle-strengthening activity must push the muscle to its limit. This is the only message it will respond to. But how you get there is up to you. You can do it quickly with a few repetitions of a large weight, or you can do it slowly with many repetitions of a more bearable weight. The first method builds bulk fast—especially for men. The second takes time and builds lean, strong muscles that are firm and shapely but not particularly large. Keep in mind that bone seems to respond better to a few repetitions of a heavy load than to many repetitions of a smaller one.

Whole-Body Workout

Weight training is very specific. For example, lifting weights with your left arm will only benefit your left arm. If you want to use exercise to counter bone loss, you must work out your whole body. If you already spend plenty of time on your feet, you might begin by focusing on your upper body.

There are over six hundred skeletal muscles in the human body, but a complete regimen is generally encompassed by systematically working out the legs, lower back, chest, upper back, arms and shoulders. A good trainer will show you the meaning and importance of good form by example, and will take into account your state of health, any injuries you may have, and your level of motivation. You can hurt yourself with weights if you're not careful, and an injury early on in a new program could turn you off exercise for life. So be careful, and consult a good trainer at the beginning and at least once in a while thereafter. Above all, learn to listen carefully to your body before, during, and after the workout. It may creak and ache a little, but it will also thank you as it grows stronger.

THE DANGERS OF OVEREXERCISE

You can train too much. If you've worked out or lifted sensible weights without overstraining yourself, your muscles will ache a little, more if you haven't worked muscles in a long time. After a workout, give your muscles the time they need to recover. Doctors recommend at least forty-eight hours, but professional fitness trainers have devised a variety of ingenious ways to trick the body into bulking up. The key is to pay attention to your body and to push it to its limits, but not beyond. Professional or highly competitive amateur athletes are often driven by goals other than long-term health. In addition, young men—and increasingly young women—are driven by the desire to improve the appearance of their bodies. This often leads them to focus on the more cosmetic muscles such as the pectorals (chest muscles), which rarely require great strength in daily life, even for manual workers. If you are exercising for your health, your routines will be more moderate and should focus on the areas that count most—the abdominal and back muscles that are crucial to good posture, and the lower body muscles that keep you on your feet.

The overtrained athlete experiences a host of physiological effects that inevitably lead to poor performance and eventual illness. They include fluctuations in insulin secretion, alterations in glucocorticoid and hormone levels, inhibition of glucose uptake to tissues, catabolic (breakdown) effects on protein and nitrogen excretion, and lactic acid overproduction. In women, overexercise can interfere with menstrual regularity, affecting estrogen secretion and possibly increasing bone loss. Some women develop amenorrhea (complete cessation of menstrual periods). They are risking early bone loss comparable to that experienced during normal menopause. Just one or two years of this condition at an early age can be disastrous.

If you are on any medication or have any injuries or weaknesses that might inhibit your cardiovascular performance or ability to lift weights—such as existing osteopenia or osteoporosis—you should consult your physician and/or a physiotherapist before embarking on any sort of strenuous exercise regimen.

Preventing Falls

While vertebral fractures are commonly caused by the crushing effect of body weight upon the spine or by an otherwise routine movement, osteoporotic fractures in other bones are usually caused by falls. Elderly people with weakened bones are at greatest risk. Declining vision, poor coordination, muscular weakness, and inflexibility all contribute to falls. Some medications can cause drowsiness, dizziness, impaired balance, and distraction. Canes or walkers can help minimize dangers, but many people reject these visible signs of weakness until they experience a trauma and find they have no choice. A whole industry has grown up around fall-saving devices.

Most falls occur at home. The bathroom is the most dangerous room. Well-situated grab bars around the tub and rubber matting inside it will help you during the most precarious movements—stepping in and out, and lowering and raising yourself from the water. If you have trouble sitting down in the bath, a bath bench or chair may be useful. You can also purchase a transfer bench, which extends over the edge and enables you to safely maneuver your legs over the tub.

If you get up in the night, make sure your path is clear and well lit. Of all times of day, this is when people need to pay close attention to their steps. Night-lights help. Movement-activated lights are even better.

Avoid washing or polishing your floors with anything that makes them slippery. Beware of area rugs that might easily slide underfoot or catch your toes and trip you. Above all, wear comfortable shoes that hold your foot well, give all-around support, and have short wide heels and nonslip soles.

And when you step out of the house, keep your eyes firmly on the path ahead of you. A small bump or crack in the pavement can lead to a very moderate fall but cause an injury that might lay you up for months or even years. A large portion of fall victims describe their experience as "stupid" and cannot stop thinking about how easily it might have been avoided, if only . . .

Diet

A balanced diet high in vitamins and minerals is always important, critically so in infancy and childhood. We have learned that too much protein can release calcium from bone and increase calcium excretion. So go easy on meat—the most concentrated protein in most people's diet. Cheese is a good alternative that also happens to be loaded with calcium. Plenty of fruits and vegetables are as important for your bones as for the rest of your body. Junk food is best avoided but if you must eat it, at least don't let it stop you from eating fresh foods too. Despite their fondness for carbonated drinks, teenagers should keep up their milk consumption. Take calcium supplements in small doses with meals, drink plenty of water, and make sure you don't take too much vitamin A or D.

Weight-loss diets can be a problem if they are not carefully planned. Young women in particular may be subject to eating disorders that cause not only weight loss but also serious vitamin and mineral deficiencies that are extremely damaging to the entire metabolism, including bones. These disorders should not be underestimated; they are very dangerous. Any sort of nutritional deficiency during childhood or adolescence can have profound long-term consequences.

VITAMINS

Vitamins are crucial to countless metabolic functions, including the absorption of calcium and the maintenance of osteoblast and osteoclast activity.

Vitamin B

Vitamin B_{12} has been associated with the function of osteoblasts (bone-making cells). It is unlikely that you are short of this vitamin unless you adhere to a strict vegetarian diet. People who have undergone surgical removal of all or part of the stomach and intestines may suffer deficiency of this vitamin. A daily supplement is sufficient to correct the problem.

Vitamin K

Vitamin K is needed in the extracellular matrix of bone where it plays a part in the formation of osteocalcin, a bone protein. The role of osteocalcin is not clear but it seems to be involved in bone resorption. Vitamin K is found readily in green leafy vegetables and is also manufactured by our bodies. If you eat a cupful of lettuce or other greens each day, vitamin K supplementation is unnecessary. In excessive amounts, laboratory-synthesized vitamin K can cause jaundice (yellowing of the skin).

Vitamin C

Vitamin C is important in the production of collagen, a fiber that forms the matrix on which bone is built. However, deficiency is likely to cause other, more noticeable health problems before bone health is seriously affected. Scurvy is the best known disease of vitamin C deficiency. Cases of vitamin C deficiency are now extremely rare in the Western world. Vitamin C megadosing (taking several grams per day) is not uncommon, although the benefits of this practice are inconclusive. Some reports suggest that large quantities of vitamin C may result in kidney stones—an excruciatingly painful problem.

Vitamin A

Vitamin A is critical to skeletal development. It is found abundantly in green vegetables, milk, butter, and cheese. Too much vitamin A is toxic and poses real dangers. Reports of certain anticancer properties have been taken out of context, and many people have eagerly overdosed on it. Symptoms are weakness, fatigue, emotional disturbance, and aching of the head, muscles, and bones. There is rarely any need to supplement vitamin A.

MINERALS

A variety of minerals and trace elements is important to healthy metabolism, and bone itself is a predominantly mineral construction. The following minerals have been implicated directly or indirectly in the development and maintenance of bone mass. As you will see, coming to a clear conclusion about the advantages or disadvantages of some minerals is not easy.

Calcium

The mineral calcium is an important component of bone and the one most critically subject to metabolic loss. Calcium is essential for muscle and nerve activity, for which reason it may be removed from bone by osteoclasts (bone-dissolving cells). If osteoblasts (bone-making cells) cannot keep up with the osteoclast activity, the result is net bone loss.

By maintaining elevated blood-calcium levels, osteoclast activity is not stimulated and the bone-renewing cycle remains in a state of equilibrium. As we age, however, it becomes increasingly difficult to absorb calcium from conventional sources. Absorption is dependant among other factors on adequate levels of Vitamin D.

Magnesium

Recent research suggests that the magnesium in bones—just like the calcium—is used as a reservoir by the body. When there is not enough dietary magnesium, the body takes what it needs from bone. According to studies carried out at the Veterans Administration Medical Center in Loma Linda, California, magnesium supplements appear to increase bone mass in women with magnesium deficiencies—even those with osteoporosis. Other tests on young men with adequate magnesium levels measured markers in their blood for bone breakdown, and found that those who took daily magnesium supplements showed signs of reduced bone loss, suggesting that magnesium supplementation might play a preventive role.

Zinc

Zinc deficiency definitely causes disease, including stunted growth and defective production of proteins, but deficiency of this mineral is considered rare. It is present in small amounts in all types of food. It is also a significant constituent of bone. Increased zinc levels in the urine are used sometimes as a marker for bone loss, and low blood-zinc levels are typical of osteoporotic patients. Whether supplementation is in any way useful or advisable is unclear, but seems unlikely.

Manganese

Manganese is a trace element present in many foods and unlikely to be deficient in many diets. It appears to be critical to the development of cartilage and bone. The few people known to suffer from manganese deficiency also tended to be deficient in other minerals, but were particularly susceptible to bone loss and osteoporosis. Manganese is a trace element, meaning that it is only required in very small amounts. In fact, supplementation could easily and unnecessarily raise manganese levels to excess.

Copper
Diseases in which copper absorption is inhibited are clearly linked to a risk of osteoporosis. On the other hand, excessive copper seems to cause bone abnormalities. It is found in white meats and in water. Supplementation is not recommended.

Silicon and Boron
There is little evidence to support the use of silicon or boron as preventive or restorative therapies, although some alternative-health practitioners believe boron may be useful in the maintenance of bone health. The role of both in the human metabolism is so unknown that Recommended Dietary Allowances (RDA) figures have not even been determined. Further studies are needed to determine the efficacy of boron.

Fluoride
Fluoride is added to drinking water in many municipalities to combat the development of dental cavities, which it does very effectively. Fluorosis is a painful disease caused in miners by exposure to fluoride dust. It makes bones very dense, apparently by stimulating the formation of osteoblasts (bone-making cells). However, even though bone becomes denser, it does not seem to be stronger. Overall, scientists describe the effect of elevated fluoride levels on bone as deformative. While study of fluoride may lead to new treatments for bone loss, there is not enough evidence to suggest any possible role at this time.

OTHER SUPPLEMENTS
A fermented soybean product from Japan called Natto may help stop calcium loss and prevent osteoporosis, according to studies at the Kawasaki Medical School. This study was carried out on people at genetic risk for osteoporosis due to an inability to metabolize vitamin D. The soybean product had very high levels of vitamin K_2. Vita-

min K_2 deficiency has long been considered rare, but this study showed improved bone mass in those with this particular genetic predisposition to osteoporosis.

Case Study: Edward Reddy's Bones

Edward Reddy is a trainer at the Westmount YMCA in Montreal. He is just entering his seventies, and a single glance tells you he is one of the fittest people there. He's lean—not the least bit bulky—but strong. Edward's cardiologist recently described his cardiovascular performance as "ten percent off Olympic standards without correction for age." He's a tough one to beat, even for young men in their twenties and thirties.

He is also tall (six foot four) and erect. He easily pulls 130 pounds with each arm, working out his upper back one side at a time. It is evident that his strength is not only in his muscles; his bones must be tough, too, or they wouldn't keep up.

Edward's doctor wanted to know how he did it, and started quizzing him. But his answers were surprisingly inconclusive. First of all, he had only been weight-training for eight years—some forty years at least after reaching peak bone mass. He had always exercised a great deal, mostly in a variety of sports, including twenty-eight seasons of competition basketball, the last at age fifty. This sport, with its sudden, darting turns probably flexed and compressed his legs and hips considerably, stimulating bone renewal and helping maintain his youthful BMD, at least below the waist. Walking, cycling, in-line skating, and rowing probably also helped maintain his lower body. But these activities do not account for his total skeletal health because they are predominately cardiovascular workouts. Another sport he enjoys is archery. This strengthens muscles selectively but is nothing like a systematic weight training.

His diet is healthy and practical; his only supplement, a daily multivitamin. He doesn't drink alcohol and has never used glucocorticoids, anticonvulsants, or thyroid medications. He likes traditional carbohydrate-protein meal combinations (beans, a little meat, a little pasta, some fresh vegetables, no junk).

The doctor had run out of questions to ask but was still not satisfied. In spite of Edward's extremely active lifestyle, there had to be more. They turned to casual conversation. Edward chatted about his career in the petrochemical industry, from which he is now semi-retired. He had worked mostly as a foreman in an oil refinery. The doctor wondered if anything in his job description could promote such exceptional skeletal health. Edward acknowledged that he had worked predominantly in the field. "Up in the air, actually. Up and down ladders all day long," he added.

The doctor visualized a long ladder leaning against a wall, Edward using his arms to steady himself, but climbing entirely with his legs. Another lower body workout. Still, he asked him to describe the motion, which Edward mimed for him. It wasn't at all what the doctor had expected. Edward explained that they were fixed ladders, bolted to walls and perfectly vertical."

Now the doctor sat up. Edward had pushed back his chair and was miming himself climbing a vertical ladder, showing a full range of motion with his arms, shoulders, and back. Pulling his own weight vertically upward and pushing with his legs. "How often?" asked the doctor

"Oh, a three-hundred-foot ladder, at least three times a day. Maybe a thousand feet average, sometimes more."

The doctor was satisfied at last. Without knowing it, Edward had been weight-training every day at work. The weight had been his own body.

Conclusion

Prevention of bone loss begins with the identification of risk factors and a consultation with your doctor. If you have any doubts as to the health of your bones, you should get a bone-mineral density test. Whatever your current status, exercise is the first therapy you should consider. If your bones are still strong, regular impact loading or weight-bearing exercises may be sufficient to protect you. It is important to find an exercise regimen you enjoy. Be sure that your exercise regimen puts health first, rather than competition or vanity. If you are osteoporotic, take great care to minimize the danger of falling. Everybody should take calcium regularly, preferably in small doses with meals, and make sure you get enough vitamin D and not too much vitamin A. Consult the table on page 44 to review common risk factors and plan your personal approach to prevention.

7

Conclusion

Osteoporosis is a huge problem for society at large. Dr. Takuo Fujita, president of the Japan Osteopororis Foundation and director of the Calcium Research Institute, calls it: ". . . the most common disease affecting mankind at present."

Global life expectancy has risen dramatically since 1950 to its present sixty-six years, so most women worldwide live long beyond menopause, which in highly industrialized countries occurs with more than one-third of their lives yet to live. Consider also that 55 percent of people over sixty and 65 percent of eighty-year-olds are women, and that by 2050, fully one-fifth of the world's population will be over sixty. If a large portion of those people are not mobile and independent, the cost to society will be incalculable, not just in money but also in widespread physical pain, declining morale, and depression.

Incidence

Osteoporosis is a silent killer. The vast majority of those at risk either don't realize they are suffering from bone loss, or don't take it seriously because they experience no symptoms. But one of every two women and one in eight men over age fifty will have an osteoporosis-related fracture in their lifetime. According to the National Osteoporosis Foundation, this disease threatens more than 28 million Americans, one-fifth of them men. Ten million Americans have the disease today and 18 million more are estimated to be at risk due to low bone-mineral density. Unless they do something about it, many of those who live long enough will suffer a painful, difficult, and expensive conclusion to their lives.

Of the ten million Americans actually living with the disease, eight million are women and two million are men. Tens of millions more have low bone density. Statistics tell us that African-Americans are at the lowest risk of all, but they too are at risk. One in ten African-American women over age fifty has osteoporosis. Another three out of ten have sufficiently low bone density to be considered likely to develop osteoporosis. Osteoporosis threatens everybody who grows old. Bone loss usually begins at the very latest by the mid-twenties, and the first fractures may strike well before the golden years.

Cost

The National Osteoporosis Foundation estimates that the cost of managing osteoporosis in the United States in 1995 was $13.8 billion—about $38 million per day. Osteoporosis leads to more than 1.5 million fractures annually, including 300,000 hip fractures, 700,000 vertebral fractures, 250,000 wrist fractures, and 300,000 other fractures.

Treatment

Osteoporotic fractures are unlike the bone injuries suffered by people with a healthy skeleton. They take the form of a collapse rather than a fissure or clean break. The material of the bone is spirited away, leaving its structure compromised. The irony is that postfracture therapy is not so different from prefracture therapy—various combinations of drugs, hormones, calcium, and vitamin D—with the addition of a pain-management strategy. These treatments are preferable and much more effective when taken before an osteoporotic fracture than afterwards.

A good preventive regimen can minimize or stabilize bone loss, and some therapies will actually grow stronger bones. There are other advantages to prevention. Many of these approaches improve calcium absorption and minimize the secondary hyperparathyroidism of aging. This leaves parathyroid hormone levels at low or moderate levels, preventing the unmitigated flood of calcium into soft tissue and slowing the progress of other Calcium Paradox diseases.

Beginning these therapies after complications set in can help slow continued bone loss, prevent further damage, and, it is hoped, strengthen remaining undamaged bones. Technologies such as vertebroplasty are a very helpful advance—doctors are relieved to have at least something to offer people in chronic pain—but there is no substitute for healthy, living bone.

There is no doubt that in most cases, osteoporosis can be prevented. Millions of women have already escaped or delayed it by taking estrogen. Nowadays, doctors routinely introduce the subject to women as they approach the age of menopause. But the notion that this is a woman's disease is simply wrong. It is a disease that affects all people and is found in every corner of the world, among men as well as women, and among people of all races and origins.

Preventive, long-term hormone or drug therapies diminish the risk of other health threats and are often justifiable in spite of dangers and worries of their own. However, only 8 to 12 percent of women take estrogen replacement therapy long enough to significantly alter their risk of osteoporosis, and avoiding bone loss is only one of several motives. Most—77 percent—take it principally to control the short-term effects of menopause, such as hot flashes and sleeplessness. Those at risk of heart disease may also benefit. Of those who quit prematurely, 34 percent cite bleeding complications, 14 percent experience weight gain, and 12 percent feel that their symptoms were unchanged or not adequately addressed. In other words, in the absence of symptomatic relief or, even worse, in the presence of side effects, it is difficult to maintain motivation.

Greater effort is required to inform both women and men of the risk of osteoporosis. Estrogen replacement holds some immediate attraction for women, but men are less inclined to consider long-term therapy against a problem they can neither see nor feel. Convincing them to engage in—and especially to continue—therapies for the rest of their lives without any noticeable feedback or gratification may be difficult.

The New Health Care

The attitude of the general population toward health-care resources is changing. Doctors are seen less and less as arcane practitioners of a mysterious science and increasingly as professional consultants who can help us make informed decisions in the face of a bewildering array of research findings and therapies. At the same time, we are being increasingly encouraged to take part in our own health decisions. When it comes to bone loss and osteoporosis, this means weighing various risk factors against one another. For example, many women are reluctant to begin hormone replacement therapy because of their fear of breast cancer. However, breast cancer accounts for only 4 percent of women's deaths per year, whereas heart attacks account for 53 percent of women's deaths per year—a figure that may be greatly diminished by HRT. And osteoporosis can kill, too—another 6 percent die following the complications of hip fracture. So in general, hormone replacement therapy minimizes the overall risk of disease. But you must evaluate your personal risk factors and make sure the therapy you choose is both appropriate and adequate. For some, a vigorous exercise schedule may be enough. Others may require estrogen replacement therapy or a regimen of SERMs or bisphosphonates.

Now, with a new understanding of the sophisticated role of calcium, new therapies such as triple-A calcium promise to stabilize the bone renewal cycle just as well as hormone replacement therapy while minimizing the threat of other Calcium Paradox diseases.

Statistical Facts about Osteoporosis

- Women can lose up to 20 percent of their bone mass in the five to seven years after menopause.
- The most typical sites of fractures related to osteoporosis are the hip, spine, wrist, and ribs, although the disease can affect any bone in the body.
- The rate of hip fractures is two to three times higher in women than men; however the number of men who die within one year of the fracture is nearly twice as high as that of women.
- A woman's risk of hip fracture is equal to her combined risk of breast, uterine, and ovarian cancer.
- In 1991, about 300,000 Americans aged forty-five and over were admitted to hospitals with hip fractures. Osteoporosis was the underlying cause of most of these injuries.
- An average of 24 percent of hip-fracture patients age fifty and over die in the year following their fracture.
- One-fourth of those who were ambulatory before their hip fracture require long-term care afterward.
- White women age sixty-five or older have twice the incidence of fractures as African-American women of the same age.

Osteoporosis on the Internet

The following Web sites provides up-to-the-minute information on many aspects of osteoporosis.

- The National Osteoporosis Foundation (www.nof.org)
- Osteoporose Stichting of Germany (www.medibyte.org/osteoporose)
- Osteovision (www.osteovision.ch)
- U.K. Department of Health (www.open.gov.uk)

- The American Society for Bone and Mineral Research (ASBMR) (www.asbmr.org)
- The Bone and Tooth Society of England (www.bonejointdecade.org)
- The International Bone and Mineral Society (www.ibmsonline.org)
- The International Society for Clinical Densitometry (www.ucl.ac.uk/medicine/bmc)
- The Lunar Corporation (www.obgyn.net)
- The National Institute of Arthritis and Muscoskeletal and Skin Diseases (www.nih.gov/niams)
- The National Osteoporosis Society of England (www.nos.org.uk)
- The Osteogenesis Imperfecta Federation Europe (www.phys.tue.nl/oife)
- The Osteogenesis Imperfecta Foundation (www.oif.org)
- The Osteoporosis Society of Canada (www.osteoporosis.ca)
- The Paget Foundation (www.paget.org)
- Foundation for Osteoporosis Research and Education (www.FORE.org)
- USA Osteoporosis and Related Bone Diseases National Resource Centre (www.osteo.org)
- The European Foundation for Osteoporosis (www.effo.org)

All statistics presented in this chapter are taken from the National Osteoporosis Foundation of the USA, 1999.

References

Chapter 1

American Association of Clinical Endocrinologists. AACE clinical practice guidelines for the prevention and treatment of postmenopausal osteoporosis. *Endocrine Practice* (1996) 2:157–71.

Bonnick, S. L. *The Osteoporosis Handbook: Every Woman's Guide to Prevention and Treatment.* Taylor Publishing Company 1997 ISBN 0-87833-843-8.

Eastell, R. Treatment of postmenopausal osteoporosis. *N Engl J Med* (1998) 338:736–46.

Gallup Organization, Inc. Physicians' knowledge and experience with osteoporosis: Conducted for the National Osteoporosis Foundation Princeton, New Jersey. Gallup Organization, Inc. (1991.)

Lane, N. E. *The Osteoporosis Book: A Guide for Patients and Their Families.* Oxford University Press, 1998. ISBN 0-19-511602-X.

Lindsay, R., Meunier, P. J. Osteoporosis: Review of the evidence for prevention, diagnosis and treatment and cost-effectiveness analysis. *Osteoporos Int* (1998) 8(suppl 4):S1–S88.

Looker, A. C., Johnston, C. C., Wahner, H. W., et al. Prevalence of low femoral bone density in older U.S. adults from NHANES III. *J Bone Miner Res* (1997) 12:1761–8.

Melton, L. J., Chrischilles, E. A., Cooper, C., Lane, A. W., Riggs, B. L. How many women have osteoporosis? *J Bone Miner Res.* 1992:7:1005–10.

Melton, L. J., Riggs, B. L. Epidemiology of age-related fractures. Avioli, L. V., ed. *The Osteoporotic Syndrome.* New York, NY: Grune & Stratton (1983) 45–72.

National Osteoporosis Foundation. *Physician's Guide to Prevention and Treatment of Osteoporosis.* National Osteoporosis Foundation; Washington, D.C.: 1998:1–38.

Riggs, B. L., Melton, L. J. Involutional osteoporosis. *N Engl J Med* (1986) 314:1676–86.

Robbins, J. *Diet for a New America.* Stillpoint Publishing (1987) 189–99.

Chapter 2.

Akesson, K., Vergnaud, P., Gineyts, E., Delmas, P. D., Obrant, K. J. Impairment of bone turnover in elderly women with hip fracture. *Calcif Tissue Int* (1993) 53:162–69.

Albright, F., Burnett, C. H., Cope, O., et al. Acute atrophy of bone (osteoporosis) simulating hyperparathyroidism. *J Clin Endocrinol Metab* (1941) 1:711–16.

Barrett, C. E., Chang, J. C., Edelstein, S. L. Coffee-associated osteoporosis offset by daily milk consumption. The Rancho Bernardo Study. *JAMA* (1994) 271(4):280–3.

Bikle, D., et al. Alcohol-Induced Bone Disease: Relationship to Age and Parathyroid Hormone Levels. *Alcohol Clin Exp Res* 17, no. 3 (June 1993): 690–5.

Boonen, S., Aerssens, J., Dequeker, J. Age-related endocrine deficiencies and fractures of the proximal femur, II: implications of vitamin D deficiency in the elderly. *J Endocrinol* (1996) 149:13–17.

Carey, V. J., Walters, E. E., Colditz, G. A., et al. Body fat distribution and risk of non–insulin-dependent diabetes mellitus in women (for the Nurses' Health Study). *Am J Epidemiol* (1997) 145:614–19.

Chapuy, M. C., Preziosi, P., Maamer, M., et al. Prevalence of vitamin D insufficiency in an adult normal population. *Osteoporos Int* (1997) 7:439–43.

Chon, K. S., et al. Alcoholism-associated spinal and femoral bone loss in abstinent male alcoholics, as measured by dual X-ray absorptiometry. *Skeletal Radiology* 21, no. 7 (1992) 431–6.

Crilly, R. G., et al. Bone histomorphometry, bone mass, and related parameters in alcoholic males. *Calcif Tissue Int* 43, no. 5 (Nov 1988) 269–76.

Cummings, S. R., Nevitt, M. C., Browner, W. S., et al. Risk factors for hip fracture in white women. *N Engl J Med* (1995) 332:767–73.

Diamond T., et al. Ethanol Reduces Bone Formation and May Cause Osteoporosis. *American Journal of Medicine* 86, no. 3 (March 1989) 282–8.

Diez, A., et al. Alcohol-induced bone disease in the absence of severe chronic liver damage. *J Bone Miner Res* 9, no. 6 (Jun 1994) 825–31.

El-Hajj, F. G., Testa, M. S., Angell, J. E., Porrino, N., LeBoff, M. S. Reproducibility of DXA absorptiometry—a model for bone loss estimates. *J Bone Miner Res* (1995) 10:1004–14.

Felson, D. T., et al. Alcohol consumption and hip fractures: The Framingham study. *American Journal of Epidemiology* 128, no. 5 (Nov 1988) 1102–10.

———. Alcohol intake and bone mineral density in elderly men and women—the Framingham study. *Am J Epidemiol* 142, no. 5 (Sept 1995) 485–92.

Finkelstein, J. S., Klibanski, A., Neer, R. M., et al. Increases in bone density during treatment of men with idiopathic hypogonadotropic hypogonadism. *J Clin Endocrinol Metab* (1989) 69:776–83.

Garnero, P., Sornay-Rendu, E., Chapuy, M., Delmas, P. D. Increased bone turnover in late menopausal women is a major determinant of osteoporosis. *J Bone Miner Res* (1996) 11:337–49.

Gonzalez-Calvin J. L., et al. Mineral metabolism, osteoblastic function and bone mass in chronic alcoholism. *Alcohol and Alcoholism* 28, no. 5 (Sept 1993) 571–9.

Greenspan, S. L., Maitland, L. A., Myers, E. R., Krasnow, M. B., Kido, T. H. Femoral bone loss progresses with age. *J Bone Miner Res* (1994) 9:1959–65.

Greenspan, S. L., Myers, E. R., Maitland, L. A., Resnick, N. M., Hayes, W. C. Fall severity and bone mineral density as risk factors for hip fracture in ambulatory elderly. *JAMA* (1994) 271:128–33.

Grisso, J. A., Kelsey, J. L., Strom, B. L., et al. Risk factors for falls as a cause of hip fracture in women. *N Engl J Med* (1991) 324:1326–31.

Gundberg, C. M., Grant, F. D., Conlin, P. R., et al. Acute changes in serum osteocalcin during induced hypocalcemia in humans. *J Clin Endocrinol Metab* (1991) 72:438–43.

Guthrie, J., Garamszegi, C., Dudley, E., Dennerstein, L., Green, A., MacLennan, A., Burger, H. Hormone therapy use in Australian-born women: A longitudinal study. *MJA* (1999) 171: 358–61.

Hasling, C., et al. Calcium metabolism in postmenopausal osteoporotic women is determined by dietary calcium and coffee intake. *J Nutr* (1992) 1119–26.

Heaney, R. P., Recker, R. R. Determinants of endogenous fecal calcium in healthy women. *J Bone Miner Res* (1994) 9(10):1621–7.

———. Effects of nitrogen, phosphorus, and caffeine on calcium balance in woman. *J Lab Clin Med* (1982) 299:46–55.

Hemenway, D., et al. Fractures and lifestyle: Effect of cigarette smoking, alcohol intake, and relative weight on the risk of hip and forearm fractures in middle-aged women. *American Journal of Public Health* 78, no. 12 (Dec 1988) 1554–8.

Holbrook, T. L., Barrett-Connor, E. A. Prospective Study of Alcohol Consumption and Bone Mineral Density. *BMJ* 306, no. 6891 (Jun 1993) 1506–9.

Johnston, C. C., Melton, L. J., Lindsay, R., Eddy, D. M. Clinical indications for bone mass measurements: A report from the Scientific Advisory Board of the National Osteoporosis Foundation. *J Bone Miner Res* 1989;4 (suppl 2):1–28.

Kado, E. M., Browner, W. S., Palermo, L., et al. Vertebral fractures and mortality in older women. *Arch Intern Med* (1999) 159:1215–20.

Kamel, S., Brazier, M., Picard, C., et al. Urinary excretion of pyridinolines crosslinks measured by immunoassay and HPLC techniques in normal subjects and in elderly patients with vitamin D deficiency. *Bone Miner* (1994) 26:197–208.

Kanis, J. A., Melton, III, L. J., Christiansen, C., Johnston, C. C., Khaltaev, N. The diagnosis of osteoporosis. *J Bone Miner Res* (1994) 9:1137.

Khosla, S., Atkinson, E. J., Melton, III, L. J., Riggs, B. L. Effects of age and estrogen status on serum parathyroid hormone levels and biochemical markers of bone turnover in women—a population-based study. *J Clin Endocrinol Metab* (1997) 82:1522–27.

Klein, R. F. Alcohol-Induced bone disease: impact of ethanol on osteoblast proliferation. *Alcohol Clin Exp Res* 21, no. 3 (May 1997) 392–9.

Laitinen, K., et al. Bone mineral density and abstention-induced changes in bone and mineral metabolism in noncirrhotic male alcoholics. *American Journal of Medicine* 93, no. 6 (Dec 1992) 642–50.

Laitinen, K., et al. Effects of 3 weeks' moderate alcohol intake on bone and mineral metabolism in normal men. *Bone Miner* 13, no. 2 (May 1991) 139–51.

———. Is alcohol an osteoporosis-inducing agent for young and middle-aged women? *Metabolism* 42, no. 7 (Jul 1993) 875–81.

Lazarescu, A. D., Lazarescu, D., Blut, M., Minne, H. W. *Smoking Does Diminish the HRT-Related Improvements on Biological Aging.* Clinic Der Feurstenhof and Bad Pyrmonter Institute of Clinical Osteology, Bad Pyrmont, Germany.

LeBoff, M. S., Kohlmeier, L., Hurwitz, S., Franklin, J., Wright, J., Glowacki, J. Occult vitamin D deficiency in postmenopausal U.S. women with acute hip fracture. *AMA* (1999) 281:1505–11.

Looker, A. C., Orwoll, E. S., Johnston, C. C., et al. Prevalence of low femoral bone density in older U.S. adults from NHANES III. *J Bone Miner Res* (1997) 12:1761–68.

Manolagas, S., Weinstein, R. Steroid induced osteoporosis research explains how bone loss occurs. *J Clin Invst* (July 15, 1988).

McKenna, M. J. Differences in vitamin D status between countries in young adults and the elderly. *Am J Med* (1992) 93:69–77.

MacLennan, A. H., MacLennan, A., Wenzel, S., Chambers, H. M., Eckert, K. Continuous low-dose estrogen and progestogen hormone replacement therapy: a randomised trial. *Med J Aust* (1993) 159(2):102–6.

May, H., Murphy, S., Khaw, K. T. Alcohol consumption and bone mineral density in older men. *Gerontology* 41, no. 3 (1995) 152–8.

Mazees, R. Bone Mineral Content of North Alaskan Eskimos. *Journal of Clinical Nutrition,* 27:916, 1974–7.

Melton, L. J., Atkinson, E. J., O'Fallon, W. M., Wahner, H. W., Riggs, B. L. Long-term fracture prediction by bone mineral assess at different skeletal sites. *J Bone Miner Res* (1993) 8:1227–33.

Melton, L. J., Chao, E. Y. S., Lane, J. Biochemical aspects of fractures. Riggs, B. L., Melton, L. J., eds. *Osteoporosis: Etiology, Diagnosis and Management.* Raven Press New York (1988) 111–31.

Naves, D. M., O'Neill, T. W., Silman, A. J. The influence of alcohol consumption on the risk of vertebral deformity, European Vertebral Osteoporosis Study Group. *Osteoporos Int* 7, no. 1 (1997) 65–71.

Odvina, C. V., et al. Effect of heavy alcohol intake in the absence of liver disease on bone mass in black and white men. *J Clin Endocrinol Metab* 80, no. 8 (Aug 1995) 2499–503.

Peris, P., et al. Bone mass improves in alcoholics after 2 years of abstinence. *J Bone Miner Res* 9, no. 10 (Oct 1994) 1607–12.

Peris, P., et al. Reduced spinal and femoral bone mass and deranged bone mineral metabolism in chronic alcoholics. *Alcohol and Alcoholism* 27, no. 6 (Nov 1992) 619–25.

———. Vertebral fractures and osteopenia in chronic alcoholic patients. *Calcif Tissue Int* 57, no. 2 (Aug 1995) 111–4.

Ross, P. D., He, Y.-F., Yates, A. J., et al. Body size accounts for most differences in bone density between Asian and Caucasian women. *Calcif Tissue Int* (1996) 59:339–43.

Saag, K. et al. Alendronate for the prevention and treatment of glucocorticoid-induced osteoporosis. *N Engl J Med,* no. 5 (July 30, 1988).

Slemenda, C. W., Hui, S. L., Longcope, C., Wellman, H., Johnston Jr., C. C. Predictors of bone mass in perimenopausal women: A prospective study of clinical data using photon absorptiometry. *Ann Intern Med* (1990) 112:96–101.

Smith, R. Epidemiologic Studies of Osteoporosis in Women of Puerto Rico and Southeastern Michigan. *Clin Ortho* 6 (1966) 45:32.

Thomas, M. K., Lloyd-Jones, D. M., Thadhani, R. I., et al. Hypovitaminosis D in medical inpatients. *N Engl J Med* (1998) 338:777–83.

Thyyari, P. P., Balhorn, K. E., Pease, A., Gallagher, J. C. Effect of smoking on intestinal calcium absorption and bone mineral density in elderly women. *Bone Metabolism.* Creighton University, Omaha, NE.

Tuppurainen, M., et al. Risks of perimenopausal fractures—a prospective population-based study. *Acta Obstet Gynecol Scand* 74, no. 8 (Sept 1995) 624–8.

Whiting, S. J., Anderson, D. J., Weeks, S. J. Calciuric effects of protein and potassium bicarbonate but not of sodium chloride or phosphate can be detected acutely in adult women and men. *Am J Clin Nutr* 65: 5(May 1997)1465–72.

Wyshak, G., Frisch, R. E. Carbonated beverages, dietary calcium, and dietary calcium/phosphorus ratio, and bone fractures in girls and boys. *Journal of Adolescent Health* (May 1994) 15(3):210–15.

Chapter 3

Aaron, J. E., Gallagher, J. C., Anderson, J., et al. Frequency of osteomalacia and osteoporotic fractures of the proximal femur. *Lancet* (1974) 1:229–33.

Baker, M. R., McDonald, H., Peacock, M., Nordin, B. E. C. Plasma 25-hydroxyvitamin D concentrations in patients with fractures of the femoral neck. *BMJ* (1979) 1:589.

Baran, D. T., Faulkner, K. G., Genant, H. K., Miller, P. D., Pacifici, R. Diagnosis and management of osteoporosis. *Calcif Tissue Int* (1997) 61:433–40.

Chalmers, J., Barclay, A., Davison, A. M., MacLeod, D. A. D., Williams, D. S. Quantitative measurements of osteoid in health and disease. *Clin Orthop* (1969) 63:196–209.

Cosman, F., Nieves, J., Wilkinson, C., Schnering, D., Shen, V., Lindsay, R. Bone density change and biochemical indices of skeletal turnover. *Calcif Tissue Int* (1996) 58:236–43.

Cummings, S. R., Black, D. Should perimenopausal women be screened for osteoporosis? *Ann Intern Med* (1986) 104:817–23.

Cummings, S. R., Black, D. M., Nevitt, M. C., et al. Bone density at various sites for prediction of hip fractures. *Lancet* (1993) 341:72–75.

Dawson-Hughes, B., Dalial, G. E. Effect of radiographic abnormalities on rate of bone loss from the spine. *Calcif Tissue Int* (1990) 46:280–81.

Dubin, N. H., Monahan, L. K., Yu-Yahiro, J. A., Michael, R. H., Zimmerman, S. I., Hawkes, W., Hebel, J. R., Fox, K. M., Magaziner, J. Serum concentrations of steroids, parathyroid hormone, and calcitonin in postmenopausal women during the year following hip fracture: Effect of location of fracture and age. *J Gerontol A Biol Sci Med Sci* (Sep 1999) 54(9):M467–73.

Genant, H. K., Engelke, K., Fuerst, T., et al. Noninvasive assessment of bone mineral and structure: State of the art. *J Bone Miner Res* (1996) 11:707–30.

Greenspan, S. L., Bouxsein, M. L., Melton, M. E., et al. Precision and discriminatory ability of calcaneal bone assessment technologies. *J Bone Miner Res* (1997) 12:1303–13.

Hordon, L. D., Peacock, M. Osteomalacia and osteoporosis in femoral neck fracture. *Bone Miner* (1990)11:247–59.

Huang, C., Ross, P. D., Wasnich, R. D. Short-term and long-term fracture prediction by bone mass measurements. *J Bone Miner Res* (1998) 13:107–13.

International Committee for Standards on Bone Measurement. Standardization of femur. *BMD [Letter]. J Bone Miner Res* (1997) 12:1316–7.

Johnston, C. C., Norton, J., Khairi, M. R. A., et al. Heterogeneity of fracture syndromes in postmenopausal women. *J Clin Endocrinol Metab* (1985) 61:551–56.

Kanis, J. A., and the WHO Study Group. Assessment of fracture risk and its application to screening for postmenopausal osteoporosis: Synopsis of a WHO report. *Osteoporos Int* (1994) 4:368–81.

Lips, P., Netelenbos, J. C., Jongen, M. J. M., et al. Histomorphometric profile and vitamin D status in patients with femoral neck fracture. *Metab Bone Dis Rel Res* (1982) 4:85–93.

Marshall, D., Johnell, O., Wedel H. Meta-analysis of how well measures of bone mineral density predict occurrence of osteoporotic fractures. *BMJ* (1996) 312:1254–59.

Marshall, L. A., Cain, D. F., Dmowski, W. P., Chesnut, C. H., III. Urinary N-telopeptides to monitor bone resorption while on GnRH agonist therapy. *Obstet Gynecol* (1996) 87:350–54.

Melton, L. J., Atkinson, E. J., O'Fallon, W. M., Wahner, H. W., Riggs, B. L. Long-term fracture prediction by bone mineral assessed at different skeletal sites. *J Bone Miner Res* (1993) 8:1227–33.

Orwoll, E. S., Oviatt, S. K., Mann, T. The impact of osteophytic and vascular calcifications on vertebral mineral density measurements in men. *J Clin Endocrinol Metab* (1990) 70:1202–07.

Parfitt, A. M., Chir, B., Gallagher, J. C., et al. Vitamin D and bone health in the elderly. *Am J Clin Nutr* (1982) 36:1014–31.

Ross, P. D., Davis, J. W., Epstein, R. S., et al. Pre-existing fractures in bone mass predict vertebral fracture incidence in women. *Ann Intern Med* (1991) 114:914–23.

Sokoloff, L. Occult osteomalacia in American (USA) patients with fracture of the hip. *Am J Surg Pathol* (1978) 2:21–30.

Solomon, L. Fracture of the femoral neck in the elderly: Bone aging or disease? *S Afr J Surg* (1973) 11:269–79.

World Health Organization. Assessment of fracture risk and its application to screening for postmenopausal osteoporosis. *World Health Organization Technical report series.* Geneva, Switzerland (1994).

Chapter 4

Black, D. M., Cummings, S. R., Karpf, D. B., et al, and the Fracture Intervention Trial Research Group. Randomised trial of effect of alendronate on risk of fracture in women with existing vertebral fractures. *Lancet* (1996) 348:1535–41.

———. Randomised trial of effect of alendronate on risk of fracture in women with existing vertebral fractures. *Lancet* (1996) 348:1535–41.

Bouillon, R. A., Auwerx, J. H., Lissens, W. D., Pelemans, W. K. Vitamin D status in the elderly: Seasonal substrate deficiency causes 1,25-dihydroxycholecalciferol deficiency. *Am J Clin Nutr* (1987) 45:755–63.

Carter, P. H., Juppner, H., Gardella, T. J. Studies of the N-terminal region of a parathyroid hormone-related peptide (1–36) analog: Receptor subtype-selective agonists, antagonists, and photochemical cross-linking agents. *Endocrinology* (Nov 1999) 140(11):4972–81.

Cauley, J. A., Seeley, D. G., Ensrud, K., et al. Estrogen replacement therapy and fractures in older women. *Ann Intern Med* (1995) 122:9–16.

Chapuy M. C., Arlot, M. E., Duboeuf, F., et al. Vitamin D_3 and calcium to prevent hip fractures in elderly women. *N Engl J Med* (1992) 327:1637–42.

Christiansen, C., Riis, B. J. 17 Beta-estradiol and continuous norethisterone. *J Clin Endocrinol Metab* (1990) 71:836–41.

Col, N. F., Eckman, M. H., Karas, R. H., et al. Patient-specific decisions about hormone replacement therapy in postmenopausal women. *JAMA* (1997) 277:1140–47.

Cummings, S. R., Black, D. M., Thompson, D. E., et al, for the Fracture Intervention

Trial Research Group. Effect of alendronate on risk of fracture in women with low bone density but without vertebral fractures. *JAMA* (1998) 280:2077–82.

Cummings, S. R., Eckert, S., Krueger, K. A., et al. The effect of raloxifene on risk of breast cancer in postmenopausal women. *JAMA* (1999) 281:2189–97.

Dawson-Hughes, B., Harris, S. S., Krall, E. A., Dallal, G. E. Effect of calcium and vitamin D supplementation on bone density in men and women 65 years of age and older. *N Engl J Med* (1977) 337:670–76.

Delmas, P. D., Bjarnason, N. H., Mitlak, B. H., et al. Effects of raloxifene on bone mineral density, serum cholesterol concentrations, and uterine endometrium in postmenopausal women. *N Engl J Med* (1997) 337:1641–47.

Eastell, R., Minne, H., Sorensen, O., et al. Risedronate reduces fracture risk in women with established postmenopausal osteoporosis. *Calcif Tissue Int* (1999) 64 (suppl 1):S43.

Ensrud, K., Black, D., Recker, R., et al, for the MORE Study Group. The effect of 2 and 3 years of raloxifene on vertebral and non-vertebral fractures in postmenopausal women with osteoporosis. *Bone* (1998) 23(suppl):S174.

Ettinger, B., Black, D., Cummings, S., et al. Raloxifene reduces the risk of incident vertebral fractures: 24 month interim analyses. *Osteoporos Int* (1998) 8(suppl 3):11.

Ettinger, B., Black, D. M., Mitlak, B. H., et al. Reduction of vertebral fracture risk in postmenopausal women with osteoporosis treated with raloxifene: Results from a 3-year randomized trial. *JAMA* (1999) 282:637–45.

Ettinger, B., Genant, H. K., Cann, C. E. Postmenopausal bone loss is prevented by treatment with low-dosage estrogen with calcium. *Ann Intern Med* (1987) 106:40–45.

Fujita, T., Ohgitani, S., Fujii, Y. Overnight suppression of parathyroid hormone and bone resorption markers by active absorbable algae calcium—a double blind crossover study. *Calcif Tissue Int* (1997) 60:506–12.

Fujita, T. Osteoporosis: Past, present and future. *Osteoporos Int* (1997) 7 (Suppl 3):86–89.

Genant, H. K., Baylink, D. J., Gallagher, J. C., et al. Effect of estrone sulfate on postmenopausal bone loss. *Obstet Gynecol* (1990) 76:579–84.

Genant, H. K., Lucas, H., Weiss, S., et al. for the Estratab/Osteoporosis Study Group. Low-dose esterified estrogen therapy. *Arch Intern Med* (1997) 157:2609–15.

Greenspan, S., Bankhurst, A., Bell, N., et al. Effects of alendronate and estrogen, alone or in combination, on bone mass and turnover in postmenopausal osteoporosis. *Bone* (1998) 23(suppl):S174.

Greenspan, S. L., Parker, R. A., Ferguson, L., Rosen, H. N., Maitland-Ramsey, L., Karpf, D. B. Early changes in biochemical markers of bone turnover predict the long-term response to alendronate therapy in representative elderly women: A randomized clinical trial. *J Bone Miner Res* (1998) 13:1431–38.

Haden, S., Fuleihan, G. E., Angell, J. E., Cotran, N. M., LeBoff, M. S. Calcidiol and PTH levels in women attending an osteoporosis program. *Calcif Tissue Int* (1999) 64:275–79.

Hosking, D., Chilvers, C. E. D., Christiansen, C., et al. Prevention of bone loss with alendronate in postmenopausal women under 60 years of age. *N Engl J Med* (1998) 338:485–92.

Hulley, S., Grady, D., Bush, T., et al. for the Heart and Estrogen/Progestin Replacement Study (HERS) Research Group. Randomized trial of estrogen plus progestin for secondary prevention of coronary heart disease in postmenopausal women. *JAMA* (1998) 280:605–13.

Jongen, M. J. M., VanGinkel, F. C., van der Vijgh, W. J. F., Kuiper, S., Netelenbos, J. C., Lips, P. An international comparison of vitamin D metabolite measurements. *Clin Chem* (1984) 30:399–403.

Karpf, D. B., Shapiro, D. R., Seeman, E., et al. Prevention of nonvertebral fractures by alendronate: a meta-analysis. *JAMA* (1997) 277:1159–64.

Liberman, U. A., Weiss, S. R., Broll, J., et al. and the Alendronate Phase III Osteoporosis Treatment Study Group. Effect of oral alendronate on bone mineral density and the incidence of fractures in postmenopausal osteoporosis. *N Engl J Med* (1995) 333:1437–43.

————. Effect of treatment with oral alendronate on bone mineral density and fracture incidence in postmenopausal osteoporosis. *N Engl J Med* (1995) 333:1437–43.

Lindsay, R., Hart, D. M., Clark, D. M. The minimum effective dose of estrogen for prevention of postmenopausal bone loss. *Obstet Gynecol* (1984) 63:759–63.

Lindsay, R., Tohme, J. F. Estrogen treatment of patients with osteoporosis. *Obstet Gynecol* (1990) 76:290–95.

Lindsay, R. The role of estrogen in the prevention of osteoporosis. *Endocrinol Metab Clin North Am* (1998) 27:399–409.

Lips, P., Chapuy, M. C., Dawson-Hughes, B., Pols, H. A. P. International comparison of serum 25-hydroxyvitamin D measurements. *J Bone Miner Res* (1995) 10(suppl):S49.

Lufkin, E. G., Wahner, H. W., O'Fallon, W. M., et al. Treatment of postmenopausal osteoporosis with transdermal estrogen. *Ann Intern Med* (1992) 117:1–9.

Lyritis, G. P., Tsakalakos, N., Magiasis, B., Karachalios, T., Yiatzides, A., Tsekoura, M. Analgesic effect of salmon calcitonin in osteoporotic vertebral fractures: a double-blind placebo-controlled clinical study. *Calcif Tissue Int* (1991) 49:369–72.

McClung, M., Clemmesen, B., Daifotis, A., et al. for the Alendronate Osteoporosis Prevention Study Group. Alendronate prevents postmenopausal bone loss in women without osteoporosis. *Ann Intern Med* (1998) 128:253–61.

Okazaki, R., Toriumi, M., Fukumoto, S., Miyamoto, M., Fujita, T., Tanaka, K., Takeuchi, Y. Thiazolidinediones inhibit osteoclast-like cell formation and bone resorption in vitro. *Endocrinology* (Nov 1999) 140(11):5060–5.

Overgaard, K., Hansen, M. A., Jensen, S. B., Christiansen, C. Effect of salcatonin given intranasally on bone mass and fracture rates in established osteoporosis: A dose-response study. *BMJ* (1992) 305:556–61.

Peacock, M., Selby, P. L., Francis, R. M., Brown, W. B., Hordon, L. Vitamin D deficiency, insufficiency, sufficiency, and intoxication, what do they mean? Sixth Workshop on Vitamin D. Schaefer, N. A., Grigoletti, M. G., Herrath, D. V., eds. Berlin, Germany: DeGruyter (1985) 569–70.

Prestwood, K. M., Pannullo, A. M., Kenny, A. M., Pillbeam, C. C., Raisz, L. G. The effect of a short course of calcium and vitamin D on bone turnover in older women. *Osteoporos Int* (1996) 6:314–19.

Recker, R. The effect of milk supplements on calcium metabolism, bone metabolism and calcium balance. *American Journal of Clinical Nutrition* (1985) 41:254.

Recker, R. R., Davies, K. M., Dowd, R. M., et al. The effect of low-dose continuous estrogen and progesterone therapy with calcium and vitamin D on bone in elderly women. *Ann Intern Med* (1999) 130:897–904.

Recker, R. R., Hinders, S., Davies, M. Correcting calcium nutritional deficiency prevents spine fractures in elderly women. *J Bone Miner Res* (1996) 11:1961.

Standing Committee on the Scientific Evaluation of Dietary Reference Intakes, Food and Nutrition Board, Institute of Medicine. *Dietary Reference Intakes for Calcium, Phosphorus, Magnesium, Vitamin D, and Fluoride.* National Academy Press; Washington, D.C. (1997).

Stock, J. L., Avioli, L. V., Baylink, D. J., et al. for the PROOF Study Group. Calcitonin-salmon nasal spray reduces the incidence of new vertebral fractures in postmenopausal women. *J Bone Miner Res* (1997) 12(suppl 1):S149.

Storm, T., Thamsborg, G., Sorensen, H. A., et al. Long-term treatment with intermittent cyclical etidronate. *J Bone Miner Res* (1992) 7(suppl):S177.

Storm, T., Thamsborg, G., Steiniche, T., Genant, H. K., Sorensen, O. H. Effect of intermittent cyclical etidronate therapy on bone mass and fracture rate in women with postmenopausal osteoporosis. *N Engl J Med* (1990) 322:1265–71.

Thomas, M. K., Lloyd-Jones, D. M., Thadhani, R. I., et al. Hypovitaminosis D in medical inpatients. *N Engl J Med* (1998) 338:777–83.

Watts, N., Hangartner, T., Chesnut, C., et al. Risedronate treatment prevents vertebral and non-vertebral fractures in women with postmenopausal osteoporosis. *Calcif Tissue Int* (1999) 64(suppl 1):S42.

Watts, N. B., Harris, S. T., Genant, H. K., et al. Intermittent cyclical etidronate treatment of postmenopausal osteoporosis. *N Engl J Med* (1990) 323:73–79.

Webb, A., Pillbeam, C., Hanafin, Hollick, M. An evaluation of the relative contributions of exposure to sunlight and of diet to the circulating concentrations of 25–hydroxy-vitamin D in an elderly nursing home population in Boston. *Am J Clin Nutr* (1990) 51:1075–81.

Wimalawansa, S. J. Combined therapy with estrogen and etidronate has an additive effect on bone mineral density in the hip and vertebrae: Four-year randomization study. *Am J Med* (1995) 99:36–42.

Writing Group for the PEPI Trial. Effects of hormone therapy on bone mineral density. *JAMA* (1996) 276:1389–96.

Chapter 5.

Compston, J. E., Silver, A. C., Croucher, P. I., Brown, R. C., Woodhead, J. S. Elevated serum intact parathyroid hormone levels in elderly patients with hip fracture. *Clin Endocrinol* (1989) 31:667–72.

Cummings, S. R., Browner, W. S., Bauer, D., et al. Endogenous hormones and the risk of hip and vertebral fractures among older women. *N Engl J Med* (1998) 339:733–38.

Fujita, T., Ohue, T., Fujii, Y., Miyauchi, A., Takagi, Y. Effect of calcium supplementation on bone density and parathyroid function in elderly subjects. *Miner Electrolyte Metab* (1995) 21:229–31.

———. Heated oyster shell seaweed (AAA Ca) on osteoporosis. *Caclif Tissue Int* (1996) 58:226–30.

Heaney, R. P., Recker, R. R. Determinants of endogenous fecal calcium in healthy women. *J Bone Miner Res* (1994) 9(10)1621–7.

Johnston, C. C., Jr., Miller, J. Z., Slemenda, C. W., et al. Calcium supplementation and increases in bone mineral density in children. *N Engl J Med* (1992) 327:82–87.

Lindsay, R., Nieves, J., Formica, C., et al. Randomised controlled study of effect of parathyroid hormone on vertebral-bone mass and fracture incidence among post-menopausal women on oestrogen with osteoporosis. *Lancet* (1997) 350:550–55.

Lips, P., Hackeng, W. H. L., Jongen, M. J. M., Van Ginkel, F. C., Netelenbos, J. C. Seasonal variation in serum concentrations of parathyroid hormone in elderly people. *J Clin Endocrinol Metab* (1983) 57:204–6.

Masiukiewicz, U. S., Insogna, K. L. The Role of Parathyroid Hormone in the Pathogenesis, Prevention and Treatment of Postmenopausal Osteoporosis. *Aging,* Milano (Jun 1998) 10:3, 232–9.

Nakade, O., Mandokoro, A., Koyama, H., Hattori, Y., Ariji, H., Kaku, T. *Oral Administration of Melatonin Increases Cancellous Bone Mass in Young Growing Mice.* Oral Pathology, Health Sciences University of Hokkaido, Ishikari-Tobetsu, Hokkaido, Japan. ASBMR 21st Annual Meeting Abstracts.

———. *Oral Administration of Melatonin Increases Cancellous Bone Mass in Young Growing Mice.* Oral Pathology, Health Sciences University of Hokkaido, Ishikari-Tobetsu, Hokkaido, Japan.

Ooms, M. E., Lips, P., Roos, J. C., et al. Vitamin D status and sex hormone binding globulin: determinants of bone turnover and bone mineral density in elderly women. *J Bone Miner Res* (1995) 10:1177–84.

Chapter 6

Adami, S., Gatti, D., Braga, V., Bianchini, D., Rossini, M. Site-specific effects of strength training on bone structure and geometry of ultradistal radius in postmenopausal women. *J Bone Miner Res* (1999) 14: 120–24.

Bergula, A. P., Huang, W., Frangos, J. A. Femoral vein ligation increases bone mass in the hindlimb suspended rat. *Bone* (1999) 24: 171–77.

Campbell, W. W., Joseph, L. J. O., Davey, S. L., Cyr-Campbell, D., Anderson, R. A., Evans, W. J. Effects of resistance training and chromium picolinate on body composition and skeletal muscle in older men. *J Appl Physiol* (1999) 86: 29–39.

Damilakis, J., Perisinakis, K., Kontakis, G., Vagios, E., Gourtsoyiannis, N. Effect of lifetime occupational physical activity on indices of bone mineral status in healthy postmenopausal women. *Calcif Tissue Int* (1999) 64: 112–16.

De Souza, M. J., Miller, B. E., Loucks, A. B., Luciano, A. A., Pescatello, L. S., Campbell, C. G., Lasley, B. L. High frequency of luteal phase deficiency and anovulation in recreational women runners: blunted elevation in follicle-stimulating hormone observed during luteal-follicular transition. *J Clin Endocrinol Metab* (1998) 83: 4220–32.

Emslander, H. C., Sinaki, M., Muhs, J. M., Chao, E. Y. S., Wahner, H. W., Bryant, S., Riggs, B. L., Eastell, R. Bone mass and muscle strength in female college athletes (runners and swimmers). *Mayo Clin Proc* (1998) 73: 1151–60.

Fry, A. C., Kraemer, W. J., Ramsey, L. T. Pituitary-adrenal-gonadal responses to high-intensity resistance exercise overtraining. *J Appl Physiol* (1998) 85: 2352–59.

Heinonen, A., Kannus, P., Sievanen, H., Pasanen, M., Oja, P., Vuori, I. Good maintenance of high-impact activity-induced bone gain by voluntary, unsupervised exercises: An 8-month follow-up of a randomized controlled trial. *J Bone Miner Res* (1999) 14: 125–28.

Iwamoto, J., Yeh, J. K., Aloia, J. F. Differential effect of treadmill exercise on three cancellous bone sites in the young growing rat. *Bone* (1999) 24: 163–69.

Kawata, T., Fujita, T., Tokimasa, C., Kawasoko, S., Kaku, M., Sugiyama, H., Niida, S., Tanne, K. Suspension "hypokinesia/hypodynamia" may decrease bone mass by stimulating osteoclast production in ovariectomized mice. *J Nutr Sci Vitaminol* (1998) 44: 581–90.

Kriska, A. M., Bennett, P. H. An epidemiological perspective of the relationship between physical activity and NIDDM: from activity assessment to intervention. *Diabetes Metab Rev* (1992) 8:355–72.

Lynch, N. A., Metter, E. J., Lindle, R. S., Fozard, J. L., Tobin, J. D., Roy, T. A., Fleg, J. L., Hurley, B. F. Muscle quality I: Age-associated differences between arm and leg muscle groups. *J Appl Physiol* (1999) 86:188–94.

McClung, M. R. Therapy for Fracture Prevention. *JAMA* (1999) 282:7.

Mayoux-Benhamou, M. A., Leyge, J. F., Roux, C., Revel, M. Cross-sectional study of weight-bearing activity on proximal femur bone mineral density. *Calcif Tissue Int* (1999) 64: 179–83.

Meunier, P. J., Sebert, J-L., Reginster, J-Y., et al. Fluoride salts are no better at preventing new vertebral fractures than calcium–vitamin D in postmenopausal osteoporosis. *Osteoporos Int* (1998) 8:4–12.

Osekilde, Li, Thomsen, J. S., Orhii, P. B., McCarter, R. J., Mejia, W., Kalu, D. N. Additive effect of voluntary exercise and growth hormone treatment on bone strength assessed at four different skeletal sites in an aged rat model. *Bone* (1999) 24: 71–80.

Pak, C. Y. C., Sakhaee, K., Adams-Huet, B., Piziak, V., Peterson, R. D., Poindexter, J. R. Treatment of postmenopausal osteoporosis with slow-release sodium fluoride: Final report of a randomized controlled trial. *Ann Intern Med* (1995) 123:401–8.

Pavalko, F. M., Chen, N. X., Turner, C. H., Burr, D. B., Atkinson, S., Hsieh, Y.-F., Qiu, J., Duncan, R. L. Fluid shear-induced mechanical signaling in MC3T3-E1 osteoblasts requires cytoskeleton-integrin interactions. *Am J Physiol* (1998) 275: C1591–1601.

Pettersson, U., Stalnacke, B-M., Ahlenius, G-M., Henriksson-Larsen, K., Lorentzon, R. Low bone mass density at multiple skeletal sites, including the appendicular skeleton in amenorrheic runners. *Calcif Tissue Int* (1999) 64: 117–25.

Puustjarvi, K., Nieminen, J., Rasanen, T., Hyttinen, M., Helminen, H. J., Kroger, H., Huuskonen, J., Alhava, E., Kovanen, V. Do more highly organized collagen fibrils increase bone mechanical strength in loss of mineral density after one-year running training? *J Bone Miner Res* (1999) 14: 321–29.

Riggs, B. L., Hodgson, S. F., O'Fallon, W. M., et al. Effect of fluoride treatment on the fracture rate in postmenopausal women with osteoporosis. *N Engl J Med* (1990) 322:802–9.

Sparling, P. B., Snow, T. K., Rosskopf, L. B., O'Donnell, E. M., Freedson, P. S., Byrnes, W. C. Bone mineral density and body composition of the United States Olympic women's field hockey team. *Br J Sports Med* (1998) 32: 315–18.

Tinetti, M. E., Baker, D. I., McAvay, G., et al. A multifactorial intervention to reduce the risk of falling among elderly people living in the community. *N Engl J Med* (1994) 331:821–27.

Tracy, B. L., Ivey, F. M., Hurlbut, D., Martel, G. F., Lemmer, J. T., Siegel, E. L., Metter,

E. J., Fozard, J. L., Fleg, J. L., Hurley, B. F. Muscle quality II: Effects of strength training in 65- to 75-yr-old men and women. *J Appl Physiol* (1999) 86: 195–201.

Chapter 7

Looker, A. C., Orwoll, E. S., Johnston, C. C., Jr., et al. Prevalence of low femoral bone
density in older US adults from NHANES III. *J Bone Miner Res* (1997) 12:1761–68.

Praemer, A., Furner, S., Rice, D. P. Costs of musculoskeletal conditions (In Musculoskeletal Conditions in the United States). *American Academy of Orthopaedic Surgeons,
Park Ridge, Ill* (1992) 143–70.

Ray, N. F., Chan, J. K., Thamer, M., Melton, III, L. J. Medical expenditures for the treatment of osteoporotic fractures in the United States in 1995 report from the National
Osteoporosis Foundation. *J Bone Miner Res* (1997) 12:24–35.

Glossary

AAA-calcium—Active Absorbable Algal Calcium: a highly absorbable calcium preparation

Absorb—to draw nutrients from the gastrointestinal tract into the bloodstream

Adrenal glands—a pair of small, triangular endocrine glands

Adrenal hormones—corticosteroid hormone and aldosterone; released by adrenal glands

Alendronate—a bisphosphonate

Alkaline phosphatase—a marker in the blood indicating osteoblast activity (bone formation)

Alzheimer's disease—a degenerative disorder characterized by brain shrinkage

Amenorrhea—cessation of menstrual periods

Amino acids—organic chemical compounds from which all proteins are made

Anabolic—describes a protein-building metabolic action that manufactures complex substances from simple building blocks

Anabolic steroids—synthetic hormones producing a protein-building effect, mimicking testosterone and other male hormones

Androgen—masculine sex hormone

Androstenedione—a natural steroidal hormone produced in fatty tissue where it is converted to estrogen

Angina—a strangling, constrictive pain; an abbreviation for angina pectoris, or chest pain

Antacid—over-the-counter indigestion medication

Anticoagulants—drugs used to treat abnormal blood clotting

Anticonvulsants—drugs used to prevent seizures

Antiestrogens—drugs or other compounds that minimize the negative effects of estrogen in certain tissues

Antihistamine—antiallergy medication

Antioxidants—scavenging molecules that consume free radicals

Apoptosis—programmed cell death; the self-destruction of cells

Arteriosclerosis—hardening of the arteries; a group of disorders that cause artery walls to thicken and narrow

Asthma—recurrent bouts of breathlessness of varying severity

Atherosclerosis—see Arteriosclerosis

Atrophic gastritis—age-related inflammation of the stomach lining

Atrophic vaginitis—poor or insufficient vaginal lining

Autoimmune disease—inappropriate aggression of the immune response against normal, healthy tissue and processes

Beta estradiol—a type of estrogen used in HRT

Bioactivity—the initiation of specific metabolic activity by a nutrient or other compound

Bisphosphonates—a family of compounds with an irresistible attraction to calcium; a therapy to counter bone breakdown

Blood calcium—levels of dissolved calcium in the bloodstream

Bone mineral density (BMD)—a measure of bone strength and resistance to fracture

Bone modeling—bone renewal; the process whereby old bone is broken down and new bone formed

Bone outgrowths—osteophytes; accretions of calcium around joints; a common symptom of arthritis

Bone renewal—bone modeling; the process whereby old bone is broken down and new bone formed

Bone resorption—removal of bone cells by osteoclasts

Cadaver—human corpse preserved for medical purposes

Calcitonin—hormone produced by the thyroid gland that helps control blood calcium levels by slowing bone loss

Calcitriol—the active form of vitamin D

Calcium absorption—the degree to which calcium crosses the intestinal wall into the bloodstream

Calcium carbonate—a common source of supplemental calcium

Calcium citrate—a highly absorbable source of supplemental calcium

Calcium deficiency—inadequate calcium levels in the blood

Calcium gluconate—a less common source of supplemental calcium

Calcium lactate—a less common source of supplemental calcium

Calcium Paradox—a theory of bone loss, whereby a calcium deficiency in blood leads to excessive calcium deposits in soft tissue

Calcium Paradox diseases—diseases that can be explained by the Calcium Paradox, such as osteoporosis

Calcium phosphate dibasic—an uncommon source of supplemental calcium

Cardiovascular system—the lungs, heart, and blood vessels

Cardiovascular workout—systematically raising the heart rate and maintaining it there for a predetermined number of minutes

Carotid arteries—the principal suppliers of blood to the brain

Carotid atherosclerosis—blockage of the carotid arteries; a major cause of stroke

Cartilage—a type of connective tissue made of collagen; a nonbony component of the skeleton, especially joints

Castration—removal of testicles or ovaries

Catabolic—describes a metabolic action that breaks down complex substances into simpler ones

Caucasian—originating in the Caucasus; of European ancestry

Cell—basic structural element of the body; billions in number and highly differentiated in function

Cell membrane—a double layer of fatty material and proteins constituting the outer barrier of individual cells

Cell receptor—a sort of docking bay on the surface of a cell that attracts specific molecules, enabling the cell's activity to be influenced from the outside

Chemical castration—a drug-induced suppression of testosterone production; an alternative to surgical castration as a treatment for prostate cancer

Cholesterol—an important constituent of body cells; a player in the formation of hormones and the transport of fats to various parts of the body. HDL (good) cholesterol protects against arterial disease; LDL (bad) cholesterol promotes arterial disease.

Chronic—a term describing a disorder or set of symptoms that has persisted for a long time; a disorder with no cure

Chronic inflammatory disease—persistent diseases characterized by inflammation, such as rheumatoid arthritis, and any disease causing inflammation and enlargement of the lymph glands

Circulating cholesterol—levels of cholesterol in the blood

Codeine—a morphine-derived pain medication

Collagen—a tough, fibrous protein important to the structure of bones, tendons, and connective tissue; a fiber forming the matrix on which bone is built; the main protein found in bone and skin

Collagen cross-link—a measure of bone resorption; a particular type of bone collagen that passes unchanged from the bone into the urine

Collagen type I molecule—a particular type of collagen that sometimes carries a genetic defect

Colon—the major part of the large intestine

Complementary medicine—the application of both conventional and alternative health practices

Compression fracture—a type of structural collapse usually found in spinal vertebrae resulting in shorter bones, deformation of the spine, and chronic pain

Congestive heart failure—compromised ability to pump blood

Conjugated estrogens—a type of estrogen used in HRT

Connective tissue—material holding together the various structures of the body

Constipation—infrequent and difficult passing of hard feces

Contraindications—factors in a patient's condition that make it unwise to pursue a specific therapy

Coronary artery disease—a disorder of the arteries supplying blood to the heart muscle, featuring high

PTH levels and causing oxygen starvation, pain, and tissue damage

Cortical bone—hard, outer bone

Corticosteroid medications—drugs that simulate the activity of natural corticosteroid hormones produced by the adrenal glands

Crohn's disease—a chronic inflammation in the digestive tract

Cushing's disease—abnormally high levels of corticosteroid hormones in the blood

Cystophyllum fusiforme—a type of seaweed used in the manufacture of AAA calcium

Dairy products—milk, milk products (cheese, yogurt, ice cream, etc.), and eggs

Dehydroepiandrosterone—DHEA; a testosterone precursor

Delusion—false and irrational thought taken as true

Dementia—a general decline in mental ability

Depression—feelings of sadness, hopelessness, pessimism, loss of interest in life, and reduced emotional well-being

Dexamethasone—a corticosteroid medication

DHEA—dehydroepiandrosterone; a testosterone precursor

Diabetes mellitus—an insulin disorder of the body that diminishes the ability to metabolize sugar

Diphosphonates—another name for bisphosphonates; a family of compounds with an irresistible attraction to calcium

Distress—stress beyond the body's ability to respond favorably

Diuretic drugs—potassium-sparing preparations that remove excess water from the body by increasing urination

DNA—deoxyribonucleic acid; the genetic material contained in chromosomes

Dolomite—a source of natural calcium

Dowager's hump—a curve in the upper back causing the neck and head to hang forward

Droloxifene—a type of SERM

Ehlers-danlos syndrome—an inherited collagen disorder leading to bone loss

Elemental calcium—pure calcium (Ca), apart from other elements with which it may constitute a molecule, usually a salt

Endocrine glands—glands that secrete hormones directly into the bloodstream

Endometrial cancer—cancer of the lining of the uterus

Endometrial hyperplasia—overgrowth of cells of the uterine lining

Endometriosis—displacement and growth of uterine lining tissue to the pelvic region and elsewhere

Endometrium—lining of the uterus

Endorphins—the body's own natural painkillers

ERT—estrogen replacement therapy

Estradiol—a potent estrogen

Estriol—a type of estrogen used in HRT

Estrogen—the primary female sex hormone

Estrone—a type of estrogen used in HRT

Etidronate—the first commercially available bisphosphonate

Exacerbate—to make worse

Fat—nutrient providing the body with its most concentrated form of energy

Fibrinogens—blood-clotting agents

Fibrous foods—foods containing indigestible plant material that holds water and adds bulk to the feces, aiding normal bowel function

Fluorosis—a disease that increases the number of osteoblasts and causes bone to increase in density

Follicle—a small cavity; see also Ovarian follicle

Forced menopause—menopause precipitated by a hysterectomy

Free radicals—unstable, negatively charged atoms causing cumulative damage at a cellular level; free radical destruction is being implicated in an increasing number of diseases

Gallstones—lumps of solid matter in the gallbladder, sometimes in the bile ducts

Gastrointestinal tract—the pathway of food, including the mouth, esophagus, stomach, and intestine

Genotype—genetic makeup

Glutathione—GSH; multifunctional tripeptide composed of glutamate, cysteine, and glycine, crucial to many antioxidant and detoxifying functions of the immune system

Glycine—an amino acid

GNRH agonists—gonadotropin-releasing hormone agonists; synthetic hormones resembling those released by the hypothalamus gland in the brain

Gonadotropin—hormones that stimulate activity in the gonads (ovaries and testes)

Gonadotropin-releasing hormone agonists—GNRH agonists; synthetic hormones resembling those released by the hypothalamus gland in the brain

HDL cholesterol—high density lipoprotein (good) cholesterol

Heparin—an anticoagulant used to prevent and treat abnormal blood clotting

High blood pressure—hypertension; abnormally high blood pressure even when at rest

Histidine—an amino acid

Homocysteinuria—an enzyme disorder that leads to bone abnormalities, among other things

Hormone—a chemical released by an endocrine gland into the bloodstream that affects remote tissues and other hormones in specific ways

Hormone replacement therapy—HRT; usually the combination of estrogen and progesterone or progestin

Hot flashes—a common symptom of menopause; reddening of the face, neck, and upper trunk

HRT—hormone replacement therapy, usually the combination of estrogen and progesterone

Human growth hormone—hormone produced by the pituitary gland

Hydroxyproline—a marker for the rate of bone turnover

Hypercalcemia—abnormally high calcium levels

Hyperparathyroidism—overactivity of the parathyroid glands; excess parathyroid hormone in the blood

Hyperplasia—overgrowth of cells

Hypertension—high blood pressure; abnormally high blood pressure even when at rest

Hyperthyroidism—a disorder of the thyroid gland leading to metabolic overactivity and disturbance of the body's calcium balance

Hypogonadal osteoporosis—osteoporosis caused by low testosterone levels

Hypoparathyroidism—underactivity of the parathyroid glands

Hysterectomy—surgical removal of the uterus, and sometimes also the ovaries and fallopian tubes

Ibandronate—a bisphosphonate

Idiopathic—of unknown cause

Idiopathic hypercalcinuria—unexplained high calcium urine levels

Idoxifene—a type of SERM

Immune response—activation of the immune system

Immune system—a system of cells and proteins that protect the body from potential harm

Immunoglobulin—antibody; a protein found in the blood and in tissue fluid

Impact-loading exercise—exercise movements that stimulate bone growth

Implantation—natural embedding of an egg in the lining of the uterus

Impotence—the inability to achieve or maintain a penile erection

Inert—inactive; unable to effect a metabolic response

Infection—the establishment and proliferation of a colony of bacteria, viruses, fungi, or other disease-causing microorganisms in the body, usually provoking an immune response

Inflammation—redness, swelling, heat, and pain in a tissue due to injury or infection

Inflammatory bowel disease—chronic intestinal inflammation

Insomnia—inability to sleep

Integrity—the tendency of a system or organ to maintain its structure and function

Intercellular—between cells

Intermittent—of expected occurrence but unpredictable frequency

Intervertebral—between vertebrae

Intestines—the major part of the gastrointestinal tract, reaching from the exit of the stomach to the anus

Inuit—native North Americans who inhabit the Arctic and near-Arctic regions

Isoprene—the building block of isoprenoids; a five-carbon molecule with antioxidant properties

Isoprenoid—a group of molecules containing isoprene units

Kidney stones—stones formed in the kidney from minerals and other substances precipitated from urine

Kyphosis—hunchback; excessive curvature of the upper spine

Lactose—milk sugar

Lactose-intolerance—inability to digest lactose accompanied by nausea

LDL cholesterol—low-density lipoprotein (bad) cholesterol

Leucine—an amino acid

Leukemia—cancer of white blood cells

Levothyroxine—a thyroid hormone

LHRH agonists—luteinizing hormone releasing hormone agonists; pharmaceutical preparation used to treat prostate cancer

Libido—sex drive

Liothyronine—a thyroid hormone

Liotrix—a thyroid hormone

Lithium—drug used to treat mania and manic-depression

Luteinizing hormone releasing hormone agonists—LHRH agonists; pharmaceutical preparation used to treat prostate cancer

Lymph—a milky fluid containing lymphocytes, proteins, and fats that originates from the bloodstream, bathes all bodily tissues, and is returned to the bloodstream

Lymph node—a small organ found in the pathways of lymph vessels that filters out harmful organisms from returning lymph as it reenters the blood circulation

Lymphocyte—a type of white blood cell

Lymphoma—cancer of the lymph nodes

Lymph vessels—channels that drain lymph from the intercellular spaces of body tissues back into the bloodstream

Malabsorption—difficulty absorbing nutrients

Marfan's syndrome—an inherited disorder leading to abnormalities of the skeleton

Markers—measurable biochemical evidence of a particular metabolic activity

Marrow—the soft, fatty tissue found in bone cavities and responsible for blood production

Marrow plasma cells—a type of white blood cell normally responsible for the production of immunoglobulins, which fight off infectious threats

Medroxyprogesterone acetate—a form of progestin

Megadosing—the use of vitamins and other concentrated nutrients in quantities greatly exceeding conventional recommendations

Melanoma—a type of skin cancer

Melatonin—hormone secreted by the pineal gland and thought to control daily body rhythms

Membrane—a layer of usually very thin tissue that covers a bodily surface or forms a barrier

Menopause—the cessation of menstruation

Mesgesterol acetate—a form of progestin

Metabolic disorder—a group of disorders characterized by disturbance of the body's internal chemistry

Metabolism—all the chemical processes that take place in the body; catabolic metabolism breaks down complex substances into simpler ones; anabolic metabolism manufactures complex substances from simple building blocks

Methotrexate—an anticancer drug used against lymphoma

Micronized progesterone—a form of natural, absorbable progesterone

Migraine—an intermittent disorder provoking vision disturbances, nausea, and severe, long-lasting headaches

Milk-alkalai syndrome—high calcium blood levels due to excessive intake of calcium-containing drugs and milk

Modulate—to adjust in a controlled manner

Monitor—to track the progress of a disease or therapy

Multiple myeloma—the malignant and uncontrolled proliferation of plasma cells in bone marrow

Multiple sclerosis—a progressive disease of the nervous system

Muscle contraction—the action of shortening a muscle so as to draw together the bones to which it is attached

Mutation—change in a cell's DNA

Myocardial infarction—sudden death of part of the heart muscle; a heart attack

Myopia—shortsightedness

Nasal application—method of introducing drugs through the nose

Natural product—a substance found in nature as opposed to a pharmaceutical product; also applied to substances found in nature but rendered to unnatural levels of concentration or purity

Natural progesterone—a molecule identical to the progesterone found in the human body, as opposed to progestin, a synthetic compound with effects similar to progesterone

Nerve impulses—messages passed between the brain and various parts of the body

Neurological—having to do with the brain and/or nervous system

Noninfectious disease—any illness not caused by a specific microorganism, for example osteoporosis

Norethindrone acetate—a form of progestin

Norgestrel—a form of progestin

Obesity—excessive weight

Organic compounds—all compounds containing carbon, except carbon oxides, carbon sulfides, and metal carbonates

Osteoarthritis—degeneration of joints via breakdown of cartilage and/or formation of osteophytes leading to pain, stiffness, and eventual loss of function; a Calcium Paradox disease

Osteoblast—bone-forming cell

Osteocalcin—a protein manufactured by osteoblasts

Osteoclasts—bone-breakdown cells

Osteodystrophy—a generalized bone defect caused by a metabolic disorder

Osteogenesis imperfecta—an inherited defect leading to brittle bones

Osteogenic carcinoma—malignant bone tumor(s)

Osteolytic bone disease—dissolution of bone tissue

Osteomalacia—a bone-softening disease

Osteopenia—a condition of significant pre-osteoporotic bone loss without fractures

Osteophyte—bone outgrowth; accretions of calcium around joints; a common symptom of arthritis

Osteoporosis—loss of protein matrix tissue from bone causing it to become brittle and lose structural integrity

Osteoporotic collapse—the collapse of bones under the normal weight of the body or an otherwise moderate fall

Osteoporotic fractures—the breaking and collapsing of bone due to weakened density

Outgrowths—osteophytes; bony accretions characteristic of arthritis

Ovarian follicle—cavities in the ovaries where eggs develop

Ovaries—a pair of almond-shaped glands on either side of the uterus containing numerous follicles

Overgrowth—hyperplasia; overproliferation of cells

Paget's disease—a disease common in middle-aged and elderly people disturbing the processes of bone formation

Panic attack—a period of acute anxiety, sometimes focused on the fear of death or loss of reason

Paranoia—a delusion that certain persons or events are especially connected to oneself; a colloquial term for anxiety

Parathyroid glands—a collection of pea-sized glands in the neck (surrounding the thyroid gland) that produce parathyroid hormone

Parathyroid hormone—hormone of the parathyroid gland that interacts with calcium metabolism and the bone-renewal cycle

Peak bone mass—the point in life at which an individual's skeleton reaches maximum size and density

Peer review—the rational and empirical scrutiny of published scientific reports by the scientific community at large

Percutaneous vertebroplasty—injection through the skin of plastic cement into collapsed bones (usually vertebrae)

Period—common term for the bleeding phase of the menstrual cycle

PERT—progestin/estrogen replacement therapy; also known as hormone replacement therapy (HRT)

Pharmaceutical drug—drugs designed and manufactured in pharmaceutical laboratories; popularly but erroneously considered to be fundamentally distinct from natural products

Physiology—study of the physical and chemical processes of the cells, tissues, organs, and systems of the body; the foundation of all medical science

Phytoestrogens—estrogenlike compounds derived from plant sources

Pituitary gland—the "master gland" situated in the brain that regulates and controls the activity of other endocrine glands and many body processes

Plasma—the fluid part of blood that remains when blood cells are removed

PMS—premenstrual syndrome; physical and emotional changes experienced by women in the week or two before menstruation

Poliomyelitis—polio; a virus that usually provokes only mild illness but sometimes damages the brain and spinal cord possibly leading to bodily deformation, paralysis, and death

Polymethyl-methylacrylate—a type of cement injected into the bone during percutaneous vertebroplasty

Porous—containing gaps

Postmenopausal osteoporosis—osteoporosis caused predominantly by postmenopausal estrogen loss

Precursor—building block; usually describes simple proteins that are combined by the body into more complex molecules

Prednisolone—a corticosteroid medication

Prednisone—a corticosteroid medication

Premenopausal bone loss—bone loss occurring before menopause, caused by factors other than estrogen loss

Premenstrual syndrome—PMS; various physical and emotional changes experienced by women in the week or two before menstruation

Primary hyperparathyroidism—disorder caused by overactivity of the parathyroid glands

Progesterone—after estrogen, the second female hormone produced by ovarian follicles

Progestin—synthetic progesterone

Progestin/estrogen replacement therapy—PERT; combined therapy for postmenopausal women who have not had a hysterectomy

Prognosis—probable outcome of a disease process, taking into account the effectiveness of possible therapies

Programmed cell death—apoptosis; the self-destruction of cells

Prolactin—a hormone produced by the pituitary gland that stimulates growth of the mammary glands and production of milk

Proliferation—growth

Proline—an amino acid

Prostate cancer—a malignant growth in the outer part of the prostate gland; the most common cancer of men and usually also very slow-growing

Prostheses—artificial replacement for a missing or diseased part of the body

Protein—large molecules consisting of hundreds or thousands of amino acids

Psoriasis—a chronic skin condition characterized by inflammation and scaling

Puberty—the period initiating adolescence during which secondary sexual characteristics develop

Radius—the shorter of the two long bones of the forearm

Raloxifene—a selective estrogen receptor modulator (SERM)

Receptor—a biochemical docking bay on the surface of a cell that attracts certain molecules for specific purposes; enables the cell's activity to be influenced from the outside

Regrowth—laying down of new bone by osteoblasts in pits created by osteoclasts

Renal tubular acidosis—kidney dysfunction leading to high acid levels in the blood

Renewal—the process by which old bone is broken down and new bone is built up

Replication—the division and multiplication of cells

Residronate—a bisphosphonate

Resilience—ability to withstand wear and tear

Resorption—breakdown of old bone by osteoclasts

Restorative therapies—medical interventions to correct destruction or dysfunction of any body process

Rheumatoid arthritis—severe, chronic inflammation of joints; an autoimmune disease

Rickets—a nutritional deficiency leading to the softening and weakening of bones in children

Risk factor—any cause or condition contributing to the onset and development of a disease process

Roughage—the indigestible portion of fibrous food

Salt—a compound of any acid and a base, for example sodium chloride (table salt) or calcium carbonate, one of many calcium salts

Sarcoidosis—inflammation of tissues throughout the body

Scientific study—investigation or research based on scientific principles of accounting and objectivity, open to peer review

Scurvy—a disease of vitamin C deficiency

Secondary hyperparathyroidism—excessive levels of circulating parathyroid hormone caused by low levels of blood calcium

Secondary osteoporosis—bone loss caused by a disease that does not directly affect bone metabolism, or by a pharmaceutical drug

Sedentary lifestyle—a life of little physical activity or exercise

Selective estrogen receptor modulators—SERMS; pharmaceutical, nonhormonal compounds that mimic the activity of estrogen

Senile dementia—a general decline in mental ability related to aging

Senile osteoporosis—osteoporosis of advanced age; the stage following postmenopausal osteoporosis

Serine—an amino acid

SERMs—selective estrogen receptor modulators; pharmaceutical, nonhormonal compounds that mimic the activity of estrogen

Sprue—an intestinal disorder that inhibits absorption of nutrients

Steroids—a group of drugs including both corticosteroid and anabolic steroid drugs

Stress—applied pressure

Stroke—damage to the brain caused by interruption of blood flow, not infrequently causing death

Subcutaneous—under the skin

Systemic lupus erythematosus—chronic inflammation of the connective tissue that holds body structures together

Tamoxifen—a selective estrogen receptor modulator (SERM)

Testes—testicles; source of sperm and testosterone

Testosterone—the most important of the androgen (male) hormones

Thrombophlebitis—blood clots in the legs

Thyroid gland—one of the main endocrine glands; helps regulate energy levels

Tibia—lower leg

Tissue—a collection of cells specialized to perform a specific function

Trabeculae—structural elements of inner bone

Trabecular bone—inner, spongy bone

Transdermal patch—dressing that releases a drug through the skin into the bloodstream

Tricalcium phosphate—a calcium salt

T-score—the average bone mineral density of males or females with risk factors approximately similar to your own at the age of their peak bone mass

Tyrosine—an amino acid

Urinary calcium—calcium excreted from the body in urine

Uterine fibroids—benign tumors in the uterus

Valine—an amino acid

Vegan—one who shuns all animal products, including milk

Vegetarian—one who does not eat animal flesh; some people who avoid only red meat also describe themselves as vegetarian

Vertebrae—individual bones of the spine

Vertebral compression fractures—structural collapse of vertebrae

Vertebroplasty—a mechanical treatment involving the injection of bone cement into bones damaged by compression fracture

Vitamin—a group of complex nutrients essential in small amounts to the functioning of the body

Index

ABOUT THE AUTHOR

Stephen Schettini is a journalist and medical book writer for professionals and the general public. He has written extensively on the cardiovascular system, arthritis, hormone replacement therapy, allergies and antihistamines, dermatology, and prostate cancer. He has also written *Glutathione (GSH): Your Body's Most Powerful Healing Agent*, which he co-authored with Jimmy Gutman, M.D., and he was the research consultant for *The Science Behind Squalene*, by Dr. Bikul Das. He lives in Montreal, Canada.